THE CHINA STUDY
COOKBOOK

THE CHINA STUDY
COOKBOOK

REVISED AND
EXPANDED EDITION

with Over 175 Whole Food,
Plant-Based Recipes

LeAnne Campbell, PhD

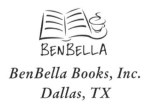

BenBella Books, Inc.
Dallas, TX

BenBella Books, Inc.
10440 N. Central Expressway, Suite 800
Dallas, TX 75231
www.benbellabooks.com
Send feedback to feedback@benbellabooks.com
BenBella is a federally registered trademark.

Printed in the United States of America
10 9 8 7 6 5 4

Library of Congress Cataloging-in-Publication Data
Names: Campbell, LeAnne, author. | Campbell, T. Colin, 1934- China study.
Title: The China study cookbook / LeAnne Campbell, PhD.
Description: Revised and expanded edition with over 175 whole food, plant-based recipes. |
    Dallas, TX : BenBella Books, Inc., [2018] | Based on T. Colin Campbell's research entitled
The China Study. | Includes index.
Identifiers: LCCN 2017056461 (print) | LCCN 2017056953 (ebook) | ISBN 9781946885302
    (electronic) | ISBN 9781944648954 (trade paper)
Subjects: LCSH: Vegan cooking. | Cooking (Natural foods) | Nutrition. | Campbell, T.
Colin,
    1934- China study. | LCGFT: Cookbooks.
Classification: LCC TX837 (ebook) | LCC TX837 .D53 2018 (print) | DDC 641.5/636—dc23
LC record available at https://lccn.loc.gov/2017056461

Front cover and recipe photography by Nicole Axworthy
Photos on pages 5, 13, 14-15, 25, 36-37, 56-57, 88-89, 128-129, 160-161, 190-191, 248-249,
and 280-281 by Louis Rodriguez
Photos on pages 6-7, 9, 21, 330 by Elaine Derby
Photo on page 17 by Steven Campbell Disla

Editing (revised and expanded edition) by Leah Wilson and Karen Wise
Copyediting by Jennifer Brett Greenstein
Proofreading by Amy Zarkos and Kimberly Broderick
Indexing by WordCo Indexing Services, Inc.
Text design by Kit Sweeney
Text composition by Aaron Edmiston and Kit Sweeney
Cover design by Emily Weigel
Printed by Versa Press

Distributed to the trade by Two Rivers Distribution, an Ingram brand
www.tworiversdistribution.com

Special discounts for bulk sales are available.
Please contact bulkorders@benbellabooks.com.

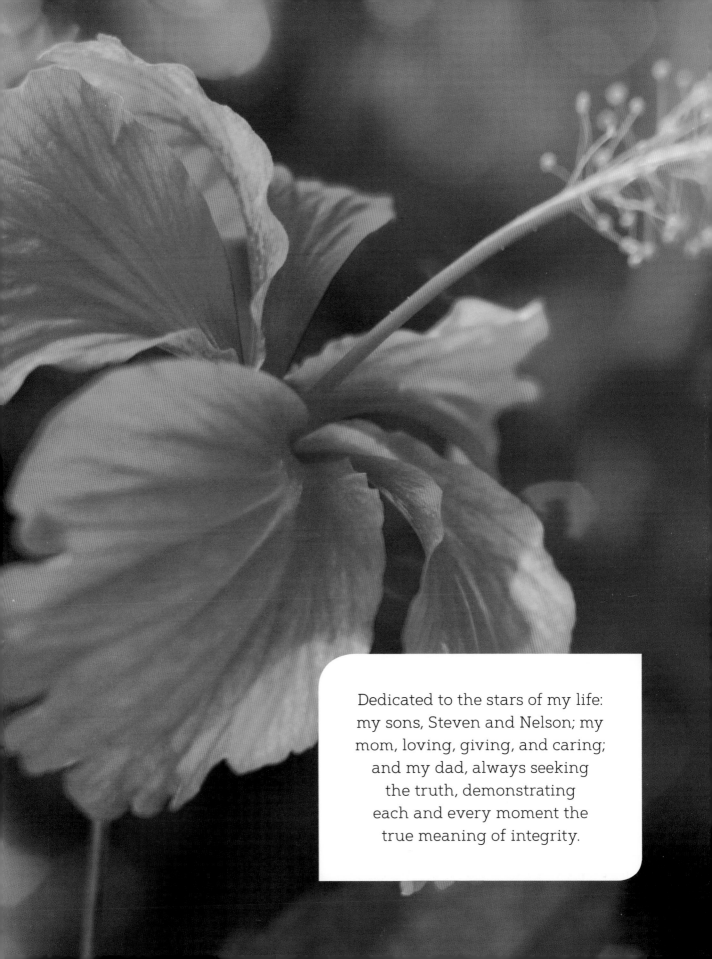

Dedicated to the stars of my life:
my sons, Steven and Nelson; my
mom, loving, giving, and caring;
and my dad, always seeking
the truth, demonstrating
each and every moment the
true meaning of integrity.

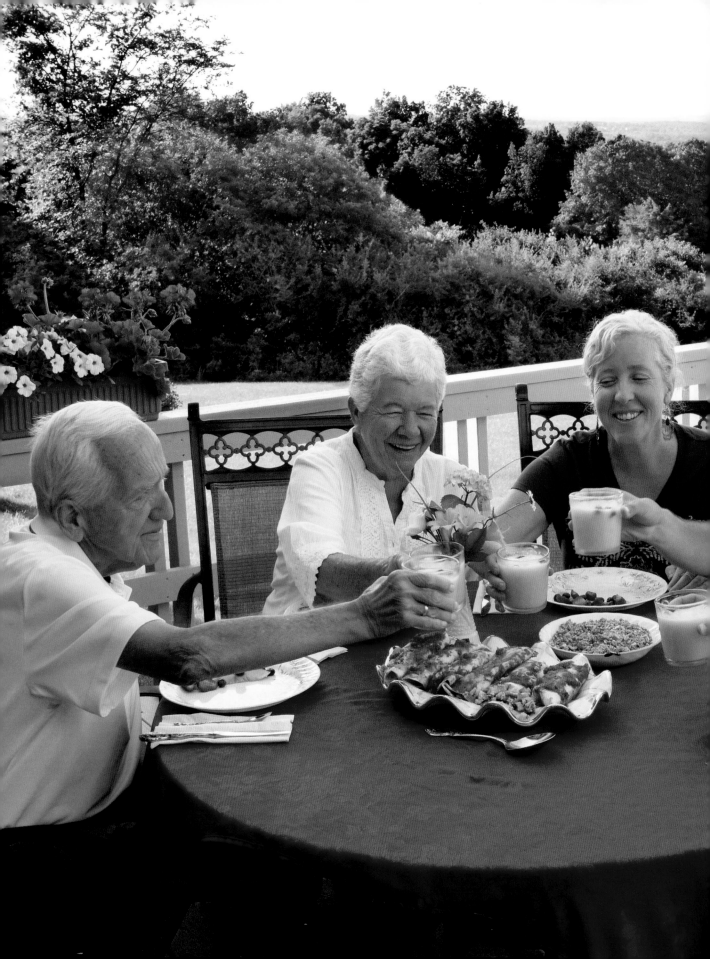

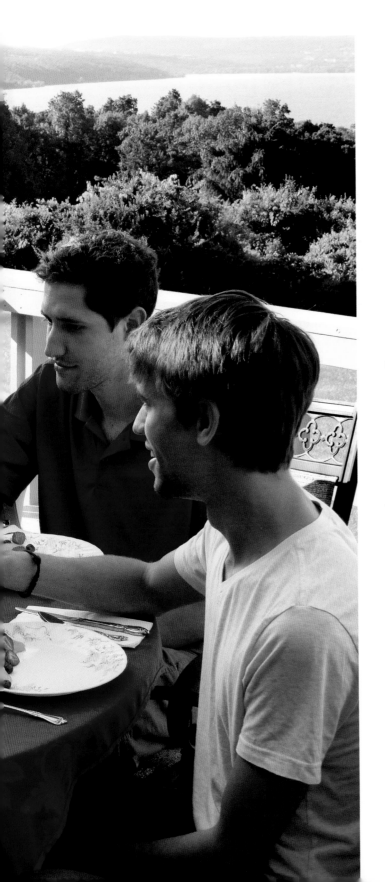

CONTENTS

FOREWORD

I AM PREJUDICED, AND I MIGHT AS WELL SAY SO UP FRONT. The author of this book is my daughter, LeAnne Campbell. But, prejudiced or not, I know her style of cooking, her recipes (I've tried many), her commitment to good nutrition, and her ability, as a very busy professional, to prepare quick, nutritious meals.

LeAnne engaged her whole family to assist with this project. Both of her sons were ready and willing to help, and they have now become good cooks in their own right. Her mother, Karen, and her sister-in-law, Kim, added a few recipes and helped with the taste testing. And I helped too—with the tasting, that is. The recipes in this book are consistent with the health message of *The China Study*, which my son, Tom, and I wrote. This book is written with the intent of helping people prepare quick, nutritious meals after a hard day's work.

One of the features of LeAnne's book is her use of recipes that contain no added fat and little or no added salt, and that make minimal, judicious use of sweetening agents. Some folks who cannot quite accept the idea of not using oil or fat in their daily diet may question her no-added-fat strategy, but the scientific evidence shows that we should try to avoid using added fat, especially those who are at high risk of getting a degenerative disease (which is most people) or who have already been diagnosed with one (e.g., cardiovascular diseases, cancers, diabetes and other metabolic disorders, and obesity). I am using the term "added" fat in order to distinguish it from whole plant-based foods that are high in fat, because the latter often contain a natural supply of antioxidants, fiber, and the right kind of protein.

I know that for many people who have always eaten the typical American diet, switching to a no-added-fat diet can be challenging—at least at first. But it's important to know that fat has been proven to be addictive, often causing people to consume increasing amounts over time. Eventually, it becomes quite difficult for many people to recover from this addiction. As with any other addiction, some people not only find it difficult to switch, but can become unusually defensive about their preferences.

Change is possible. It only takes time, perhaps as much as a few months for some individuals. And once that change is achieved, we discover new flavors among whole plant-based foods that we hardly knew existed. Once people arrive at this healthier place, many then discover that if, out of curiosity, they switch back to that old dish floating in fat, they experience some difficulties—perhaps even real intestinal disturbances—or find that the old stuff tastes more like a bad dose of grease.

I have often been asked—a few hundred times, I think: What do my family and I eat? Although I try to respond on the spot, I know well that my very limited answers cannot be satisfying to those looking to make real lifestyle changes. Now I am happy to say that there is a cookbook that comes about as close to the real deal for our family as I can imagine. This is it.

—T. Colin Campbell, PhD
coauthor of international bestseller *The China Study*
and *New York Times* bestseller *Whole*,
Professor Emeritus of Nutritional Biochemistry, Cornell University

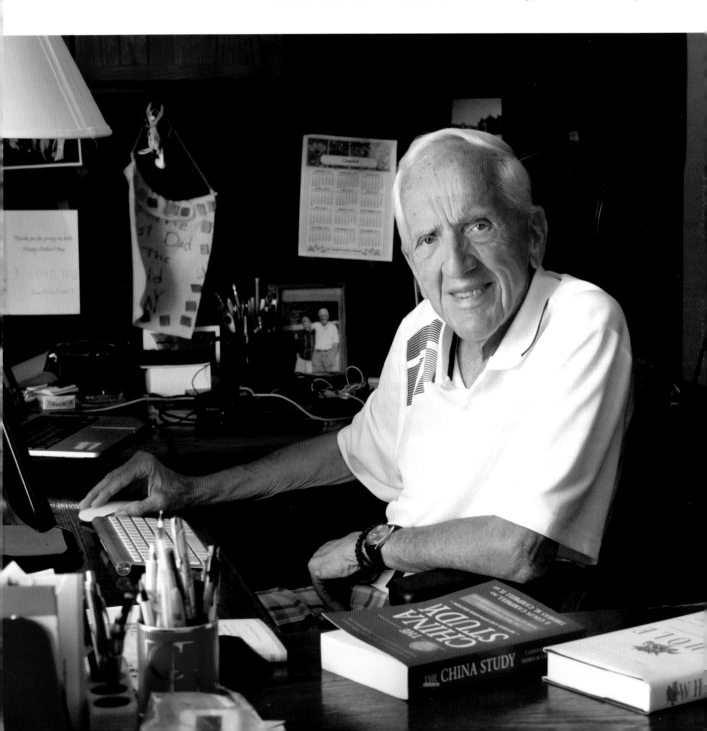

These are just some of the new recipes (many of which were inspired by the produce from my Dominican garden and from the farms in the village where I live): Mango Butter (page 47), Honeydew Ginger Smoothie (page 69), Asian Ginger Cabbage Salad (page 92), Carrot Beet Slaw (page 101), Peanut Kale Soup (page 147), Green Banana Cassava Soup (page 139), Macaroni Eggplant Soup (page 145), Golden Cheese Sauce (page 171), Black Bean Chipotle Burgers (page 164), Cabbage Rolls with Tomato Coconut Sauce (page 201), Give-Me-More Peanut Collards (page 213), Plátanos Maduros (page 267), Stuffed Eggplant with Sun-Dried Tomato Sauce (page 238), Chayote Guisado (page 259), and Passion Fruit Bliss or Black Cherry Cheese(less) Cake Delight (page 301).

I hope you enjoy them!

—LeAnne

P.S. I've created many of the recipes using the produce from our garden, including plantains, passion fruit, cacao, green bananas, chayote, black beans, eggplant, beets, mangos, cassava, coconut, peanuts, Caribbean pumpkin, batatas, tomatoes, cabbage, kale, and so much more. To see videos of these recipes, please visit our website at GlobalRoots.net.

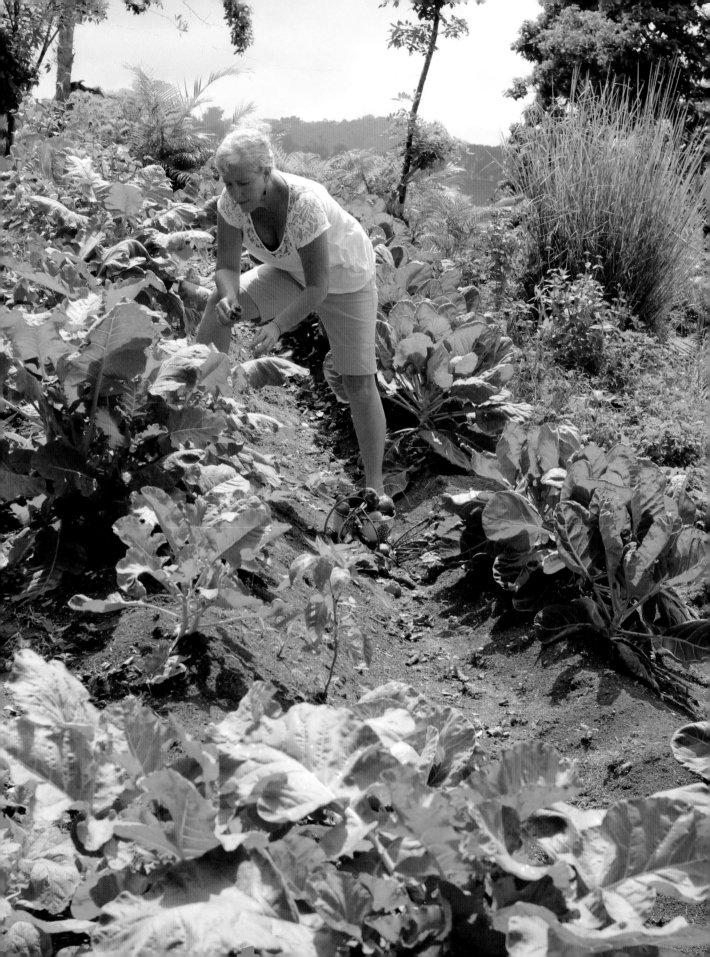

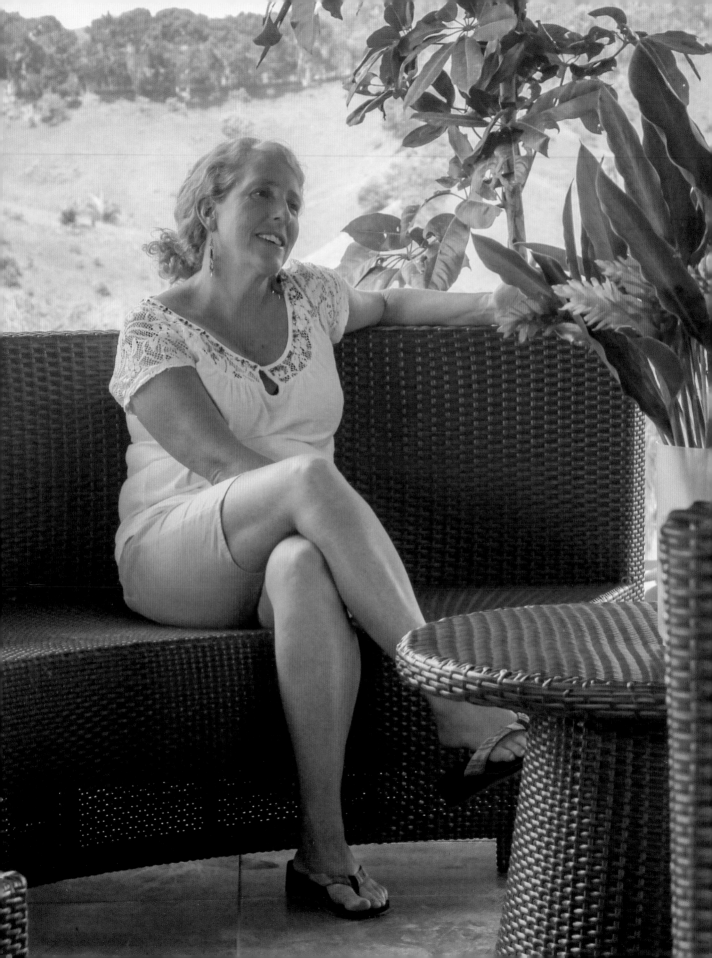

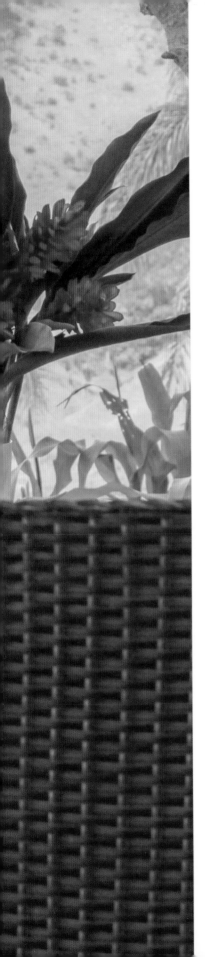

INTRODUCTION

MY JOURNEY TOWARD A PLANT-BASED DIET

WHAT YOU EAT IS A PERSONAL CHOICE, OFTEN BASED ON what you personally find tasty, satisfying, familiar, or readily available. When people ask me to think about what I eat and why I eat what I do, I have to pause for a minute. My own life experiences and those of the individuals closest to me—most notably those who cared for me as a child—have affected me, just as such experiences affect everyone. When I was a child, it was often my mother who chose the food I ate, simply because she cooked and prepared all of our family's meals. We ate these meals with gusto: pork chops served with mashed potatoes and green beans, spaghetti with meatballs, large plates of fried chicken. These dinners were often topped off with homemade desserts and ice cream.

It wasn't until my junior year in high school that our diet began to change, thanks to the findings of my father, Dr. T. Colin Campbell, which he later detailed in the internationally best-selling book *The China Study*. Based on his food-related research, he suggested to my mother that our family start following a diet centered more on plant-based foods than on animal-based foods. As a family, we slowly began transitioning toward a plant-based diet. Instead of serving meat as the main course, my mother began to use meat more sparingly, as a side dish or only for added flavor. We changed from eating a large slab of ham with a side of macaroni to having one or two slices of ham cut into small chunks and added to a large casserole dish of scalloped potatoes designed to serve eight people.

My mother was always an amazing cook, and I loved her food, so when I went away to college, I sought out the familiar, comforting foods of my childhood, which often included animal products. My college friends and I would order late-night pizza with extra cheese and sausage. We would then run down to the late-night dining hall and get ice cream sundaes smothered in hot fudge sauce. In other words, my food choices were based solely on my cravings and what I found to be tasty. It really wasn't until after college that I truly began to question why I was eating what I was eating.

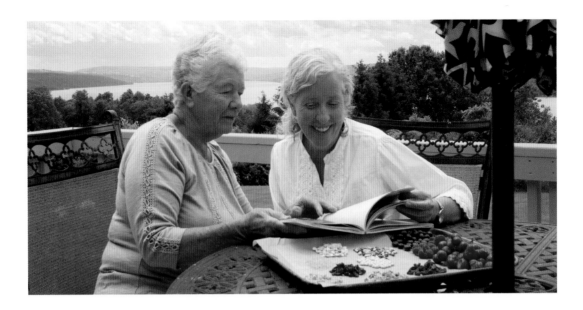

Upon graduating, I was accepted into the Peace Corps and stationed in one of the more rural areas of the Dominican Republic, one hour from where I now live. I was assigned to work directly with impoverished families and their malnourished children. There was one family in particular—and specifically one child—to whom I became attached. Anita was fourteen months old and weighed barely nine pounds. Her grandmother cared for her while her mother was in the city looking for employment, and the two often passed by the clinic where I lived and worked.

One day, I saw Anita's grandmother struggling in the rain to carry a few sacks of food that she had bought in town, as well as Anita, who had developed a bronchial infection; the two had just returned from the doctor. I offered to carry Anita. As we walked the two miles up the mountain back to Anita's home, I could feel her little heartbeat, so close to my chest. At times she was so still that I had to stop and put my ear down close to her face to hear if she was still breathing.

That evening, when I returned to the clinic, I stayed in my room. Usually I would have gone to my neighbor's house to play dominoes or just hang out in their kitchen and share stories. But that evening I wanted to be by myself. Earlier that week, I had started reading the book *Diet for a Small Planet* by Frances Moore Lappé, which discusses the humanitarian and environmental impacts of meat production, illustrating how meat production not only causes waste but also contributes to global food scarcity. And I was beginning to see examples of this all around me. Earlier that day, as I carried Anita up the mountain, I passed a thousand-acre cattle farm, the same farm I had passed several times a week for the last six months, since I was developing a community garden with families in Anita's village. The owners of this cattle farm lived abroad, and when they returned to the Dominican Republic, they stayed in their second home in a high-class tourist area. Those living around the farm never saw any benefits from this farm that occupied so much of their neighborhood. The meat from the cattle was used only to feed a small portion of the local population—those who could afford it. But those who needed it most received nothing. The comforts on

FROM *THE CHINA STUDY* . . .

Never before has there been such a mountain of empirical research supporting a whole foods, plant-based diet. Now, for example, we can obtain images of the arteries in the heart and then show conclusively, as Drs. Dean Ornish and Caldwell B. Esselstyn Jr. have done, that a whole foods, plant-based diet reverses heart disease. We now have the knowledge to understand how this actually works. Animal protein, even more than saturated fat and dietary cholesterol, raises blood cholesterol levels in experimental animals, individual humans, and entire populations. International comparisons between countries show that populations subsisting on traditional plant-based diets have far less heart disease, and studies of individuals within single populations show that those who eat more plant-based foods have not only lower cholesterol levels but also less heart disease. We now have a deep and broad range of evidence showing that a whole foods, plant-based diet is best for the heart.

Never before have we had such a depth of understanding of how diet affects cancer both on a cellular level as well as a population level. Published data show that animal protein promotes the growth of tumors. Animal protein increases the levels of a hormone, IGF-1, which is a risk factor for cancer, and diets high in casein (the main protein of cow's milk) allow more carcinogens into cells, which allows more dangerous carcinogen products to bind to DNA, which allows more mutagenic reactions that give rise to cancer cells, which allow more rapid growth of tumors once they are initially formed. Data show that a diet based on animal-based foods increases females' production of reproductive hormones over their lifetime, which may lead to breast cancer. We now have a deep and broad range of evidence showing that a whole foods, plant-based diet is best for cancer.

Never before have we had technology to measure the biomarkers associated with diabetes, and the evidence to show that blood sugar, blood cholesterol, and insulin levels improve more with a whole foods, plant-based diet than with any other treatment. Intervention studies show that when people who have Type 2 diabetes are treated with a whole foods, plant-based diet, they may reverse their disease and go off their medications. A broad range of international studies shows that Type 1 diabetes, a serious autoimmune disease, is related to cow's milk consumption and premature weaning. We now know how our autoimmune system can attack our own bodies through a process of molecular mimicry induced by animal proteins that find their way into our bloodstream. We also have tantalizing evidence linking multiple sclerosis with animal food consumption and especially dairy consumption. Dietary intervention studies have shown that diet can help slow, and perhaps even halt, multiple sclerosis. We now have a deep and broad range of evidence showing that a whole foods, plant-based diet is best for diabetes and autoimmune diseases.

Never before have we had such a broad range of evidence showing that diets containing excess animal protein can destroy our kidneys. Kidney stones arise because the consumption of animal protein creates excessive calcium and oxalate in the kidney. We know now that cataracts and age-related macular degeneration can be prevented by foods containing large amounts of antioxidants. In addition, research has shown that cognitive dysfunction, vascular dementia caused by small strokes, and Alzheimer's are all related to the food we eat. Investigations of human populations show that our risk of hip fracture and osteoporosis is made worse by diets high in animal-based foods. Animal protein leaches calcium from the bones by creating an acidic environment in the blood. We now have a deep and broad range of evidence showing that a whole foods, plant-based diet is best for our kidneys, bones, eyes, and brains.

More research can and should be done, but the idea that whole foods, plant-based diets can protect against and even treat a wide variety of chronic diseases can no longer be denied. No longer are there just a few people making claims about a plant-based diet based on their personal experience, philosophy, or the occasional supporting scientific study. Now there are hundreds of detailed, comprehensive, well-done research studies that point in the same direction.

the farm far exceeded the conditions within the homes surrounding it. The cattle had ample land to graze on. Anita, her family, and several of their neighbors lived in small, cramped quarters. Large bins of water with proper plumbing and faucets were readily available for the cattle at any time, allowing them an abundant supply of water. Anita and her family had to walk a long way to the river to obtain water, and then carry it back to their homes in gallon jugs—and even then, the water was often contaminated.

This struck me as grossly unfair, especially when I learned, five days later, that Anita had died. The cause of her death? A waterborne parasite found in contaminated river water. I was sad and I was angry. I began to question how food is produced, what resources are used, who benefits, and who does not. And I decided to reduce my consumption of animal-based foods.

I had another experience during my time in the Peace Corps that further cemented this decision: this time from an animal-rights perspective. Near the end of my Peace Corps tour, I was living one hour up the mountain from the clinic and was helping to build a school. In the field beside my house, there was a small pasture where a goat lived. This goat seemed to be rather curious and attentive to what I was doing. He often came to the fence to follow me around the yard. I started feeding him some of my kitchen scraps, undoubtedly making him even more attentive. He was the first thing I saw each morning when I went outside, and a neighbor claimed that when I returned from work, the goat would hear my motorcycle, come running to the side of the fence next to my yard, and wait for me. I became attached to the goat, who patiently waited for me each day, morning and evening.

One day after work, as I pushed my motorcycle up the backyard, I saw a slow trickle of blood. I looked toward the pasture for the goat. And there he was—dangling from the fence. His throat had been cut, and his blood was running down my yard. Yet his eyes still followed me as I pushed my motorcycle up the path. Those eyes were no longer smiling; they were pleading, begging me to help. But I could not do anything. I felt sick. I turned and went inside.

Later that evening, my neighbors brought me a plate of goat meat, telling me it was well seasoned. I could not eat it. I could not help but see his pleading eyes. This was when I stopped eating meat altogether.

I returned home from the Peace Corps with my own reasons, from both a humanitarian perspective and an animal-rights perspective, not to eat animal foods. At this time, my father was still conducting research in China. And everything he was finding suggested that from a health perspective, eliminating animal-based foods and eating a whole foods, plant-based diet was absolutely essential. Armed with my father's research and my own personal beliefs and experiences, I began consuming a diet that was close to completely plant-based: no animal, meat, or dairy products. And I've eaten a plant-based diet ever since. I now have two grown sons who have been raised on a similar diet. In feeding them, I have tried, as my mother did for me, to not only create dishes that were tasty and healthy, but use food to nourish them— including many of the dishes in the cookbook you now hold in your hands.

RAISING CHILDREN TO CONSUME A PLANT-BASED DIET

I am often asked about my experience raising my sons, from birth, on a WFPB diet. Here are some common questions I've received, followed by my answers:

Q. Do children who are raised on a plant-based diet lack any nutrients? How does this diet affect their physical and mental growth?
I have not seen any studies or research that specifically answers these questions, but based on the findings from my dad's research, I was quite confident about raising my children on a WFPB diet. If this is the optimal diet for adults, it should be the same for children and infants. And based on my experiences raising my sons from birth to their current ages—Steven is now twenty-four years old, and Nelson is now twenty-three—I would argue that they not only subsisted on this type of diet but thrived! Academically they were at the very top of their class, from kindergarten through college, receiving the highest honors possible. In addition, they were exceptional athletes, being All-State, All-Region, and All-Conference soccer players in one of the most competitive soccer states in the U.S. Steven is now six foot four and Nelson is a little over five foot eleven. Furthermore, they have rarely been sick. And throughout all of this, I never gave them supplements—I merely fed them a robust, varied, and scrumptious WFPB diet using recipes just like the ones in this book.

Q. Where do children get their calcium if they don't drink milk? What do they drink?
It's an age-old myth that you cannot get the proper amount of calcium from plant-based foods; plant foods can provide all the calcium you need. My sons use rice milk in place of cow's milk on their cereal, and in place of other dairy products in recipes, we substitute soy or almond milk. We also use these same products in plant-based desserts and ice cream. With most meals, we drink water. We try to drink at least six to eight glasses a day.

Q. How do children get enough protein if they don't eat meat?
When you consume a variety of plants, you get all the protein you need. Moreover, you will receive a *healthier* protein, since plant protein is less likely to promote cancer growth and increase blood cholesterol levels associated with heart disease.

Q. What about when children go to school? How do the other kids respond to their diet?
My sons brought their own lunches from home. Often they brought leftovers from the previous night. They would heat their meals in the morning, before going to school, and then take them in insulated containers. If there were no leftovers, they made some of the sandwiches included in this cookbook—Egg(less) Salad Sandwiches (page 169), Hummus Wraps (pages 176–177), and Granola Fruit Wraps (page 172)—plus peanut butter and jelly sandwiches.

During their elementary years, if their friends made comments about their food, my sons would occasionally make a game of it. My younger son would call his school lunch "the mystery mix" and ask his friends to guess what he was eating. The more different and strange his food appeared to be, the more he—and his friends—enjoyed the game. (One of his favorite "mystery mixes" was Dominican Rice and Beans, page 207, served with Fiesta Potato Salad, page 107, which has a bright pink tinge from the beets.) Once my sons were in high school, they no longer engaged in this game, but often their classmates would ask to taste their food and, much to their surprise, want more!

As is the case with many things in life, it was my sons' attitude toward their dietary preferences—the fact that they felt comfortable with and confident in who they were and why they ate this way—that affected how other kids responded to their eating habits. It did not matter to them that they were often in the minority or had to continuously explain to others why they ate this way. This confidence came from knowing at an early age where their food came from and the health, environmental, and social implications of their food choices.

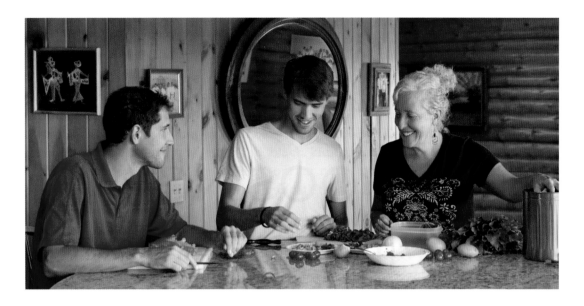

Q. What happens when children go to their friends' homes and are offered meat and/or dairy foods?

My sons' friends and their families respected my sons' dietary choices and never forced or bullied them into eating meat or dairy products. In fact, their friends' parents usually did the opposite: prepared meat- and dairy-free meals that everyone at the table could enjoy, usually a pasta dish.

When my sons traveled or went on vacation with their friends' families, I usually packed food for them to take, often rice milk and additional fruit or snacks, sometimes hummus. Their closest friends were very accommodating, stopping at fast-food restaurants where everyone could find food they would enjoy, such as Subway (where the boys ordered a vegetable sub) or somewhere they could buy burritos, such as Moe's, Chipotle, or Qdoba. Regardless of the specific restaurant, my sons were always able to order something.

Of course, occasionally my sons visited friends who didn't know what to feed them. In these instances, I made sure they ate a meal before going to the friend's house and sometimes packed additional snacks for them to take. It always worked out—even when we lived in the Deep South, where eating a WFPB diet is still rare. During the two years that we lived in Mississippi, I actually found that my sons' friends' parents there were some of the most accommodating people of all.

Q. How do you get children to eat vegetables?

I think the answer has to do with the family environment. Children will generally eat the foods that their parents eat. For instance, I don't like black olives and never use them in cooking. Neither of my sons liked olives. My sister-in-law, however, loved black olives; she cooked them all the time. As toddlers, her children ate them often.

I love a variety of plant-based foods, so when my sons were young, I always cooked different dishes with a lot of fresh vegetables, grains, and legumes. This is what they saw on a daily basis. Furthermore, I would limit the number of snacks they had before each meal, so that when they sat down to eat, they were hungry.

However, it's also important to invite children to help in the kitchen. Have them select a recipe and, if they can, prepare the dish themselves, or at least assist you. (See *The China Study Family Cookbook* for more suggestions on getting your kids involved in the kitchen.) When children prepare their own food, they are more motivated to eat it and more excited about trying something new. As we were working on the first edition of *The China Study Cookbook*, my sons helped me prepare lots of new and different dishes. And because they prepared these dishes, they were more willing to try them.

Dr. Antonia Demas, who has her PhD in education, nutrition, and anthropology from Cornell University, has done research on this. Her work shows that children who prepare their own food are more willing to eat their own dishes, even if the dishes contain vegetables that the kids previously disliked. Dr. Demas has even created a curriculum based on her research, called "Food Is Elementary" (available at www.foodstudies.org), and has used it extensively in schools across the country.

Harvesting the Garden

PREPARING DELICIOUS MEALS

IF YOU'RE LIKE ME, YOU PROBABLY DON'T HAVE MUCH time during the week to cook. I often work long hours, and when I come home, I'm exhausted. I want to cook something fast and easy. The key is to plan ahead. I've found that a small amount of time invested in menu planning weekly saves me time, energy, and money.

First, I prepare a menu for the week, trying to incorporate a wide range of plant products, including foods from the eight different plant categories. Once I have my menu, I make a list of what I need to buy in order to prepare the dishes. I buy only what's on my list, and I save shopping time by getting all my ingredients in a single weekly trip.

You don't have to plan a complex menu for every meal. The key meals are the evening ones. For dinners, I plan some simple dishes, such as slow cooker soups, and a couple of dishes that are easy to double. I generally prepare extra food each evening so we will have leftovers for the following day's lunch, and I make sure to have whole wheat or other whole grain bread or wraps and other materials for sandwiches, in case we don't have enough leftovers. Then I buy plenty of fruit for snacks during the day. One day during the week, usually Friday, is dedicated to leftovers for both lunch and dinner. Breakfasts are often the same from day to day, so I simply include some breakfast foods on my shopping list.

To plan a weekly menu, follow these steps:

1) Set aside one day a week to plan and shop for a weekly menu. I use my day off, usually Sunday.

2) In planning your menu for the week, look through your favorite WFPB cookbooks or online. There are some wonderful sites available with lots of great recipes. I generally include some of our favorite dishes as well a couple of new recipes each week.

3) Plan to make extra. I like to include five main dishes with the intent of preparing enough of each main dish to have leftovers for lunch the next day.

4) Make a list of all the ingredients you'll need for these recipes. Look in your pantry and refrigerator to see what you need to buy. Then add additional fresh vegetables for salads and side dishes, plus foods you'll need for breakfasts, lunches, and snacks (whole grain breads, whole grain cereals, fresh fruit, vegetables, popcorn, etc.).

5) Go shopping, making sure to buy only the ingredients on your list. I have found that if I go grocery shopping when I'm hungry, I buy more! So have something to eat before going to the store.

6) Keep and follow your weekly menu plan. If you don't get to prepare all your planned meals because of a workday or extracurricular event that ran late, make them at the beginning of the following week.

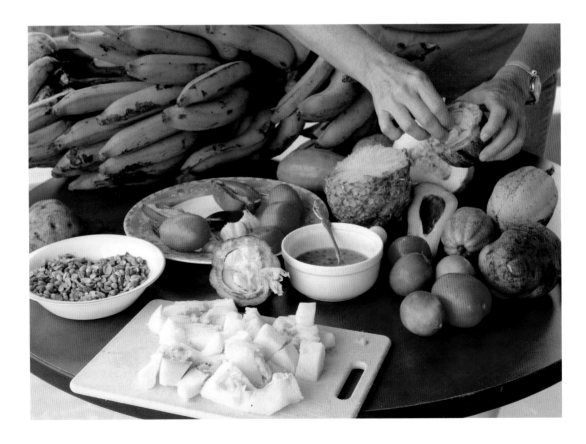

TRANSITIONING TO A WHOLE FOODS, PLANT-BASED DIET

THE FIRST STEP IN TRANSITIONING TO A PLANT-BASED diet is eliminating processed and animal-based foods.

What do I mean when I say "processed food"? Although often considered as a defined class of foods, "processed foods" does not have a reliable, settled definition. Theoretically, "processed" could mean anything from the production and initial preparation of foods to the combination of food parts to make products with special properties.

Do foods with genetic alterations count? Or foods with pesticide and herbicide contaminants? Does slicing and dicing vegetables and fruits count, as they're being exposed to air oxidation? Or, when we say processed foods, do we mean any combining of food parts (sugar, salt, fiber, oil, synthetic antioxidants) to make them tastier and easier to store, transport, or prepare count?

For this discussion, I will mostly define processed foods as food combinations having inappropriate added amounts of salt, sugar, fat, and, oftentimes, protein, as in convenience store snacks or energy-rich desserts that are high in fat and refined carbohydrates.

The definition of animal-based foods is easier: any foods that are animals or produced by animals, including meat, fish, other seafood, dairy, and eggs.

Transitioning from a diet high in animal products to a plant-based diet is a journey. There are certain foods that are made to resemble animal products,

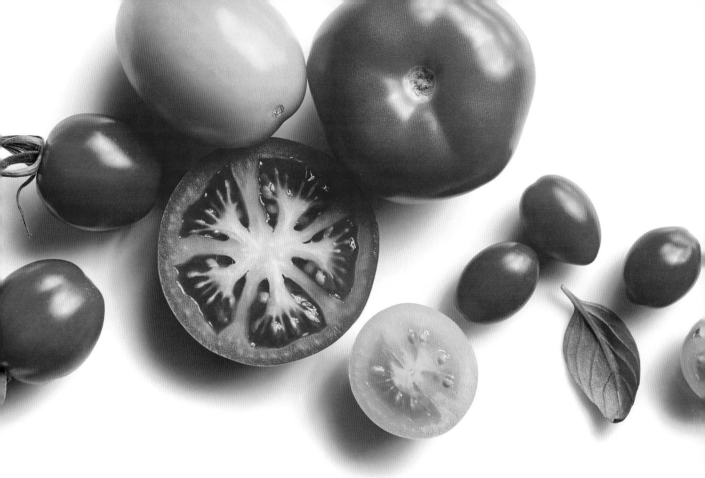

and when first transitioning, these foods can be used in animal foods' place. For instance, tofu dogs can be used to replace hot dogs, while soy-based "meat" crumbles can be used in place of ground beef. Vegan chicken and bacon substitutes are also available.

However, based on the findings of *The China Study*, I recommend selecting whole plant-based foods in their native state rather than trying to obtain specific nutrients from highly processed foods. This recommendation is based on two important points:

1) Optimal nutrition occurs when we eat food rather than use nutrient supplements.

2) The closer foods are to their native states—prepared with minimal cooking, salting, and processing—the greater the long-term health benefits.

In addition, locally and/or organically grown produce—rather than genetically modified foods or foods grown with lots of pesticides—should be chosen whenever possible.

Your ultimate goal in transitioning is to move toward a whole foods diet while choosing cooking methods, such as those noted earlier, that retain the nutritional value of the food and minimize the addition of fat, salt, and sugar. The more processed your meals are, the less healthy they are for you.

Take a look at the nutritional values of three sample lunches, ranging from fully processed to minimally processed. The differences in the nutritional breakdown are quite impressive.

COMPARISON OF THREE LUNCHES

Whole Foods Lunch

Rice and corn salad
(Corn, rice, nuts,
veggies with dressing)

An orange or banana

Less Processed Lunch

Peanut butter and
jelly sandwich

Oatmeal cookies

Orange juice

All Processed Lunch

Hot dog and bun, ketchup

Potato chips

Twinkie

Cola

COMPARISON OF THE NUTRIENT CONTENT OF THREE LUNCHES

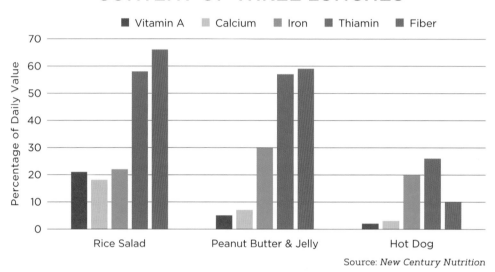

Source: *New Century Nutrition*

HOW MUCH SALT AND CHOLESTEROL IS IN YOUR LUNCH?

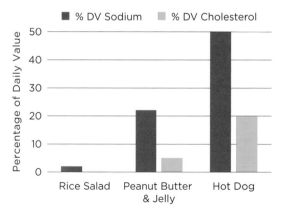

Source: *New Century Nutrition*

It's also important to think about the distinction between a whole foods, plant-based diet and a vegan and/or vegetarian diet. Why make a distinction between them? Because their nutritional content is often very different.

A vegan diet requires only that all animal products are removed. In a vegetarian diet, one still consumes dairy and eggs. And as seen in the results of a study from Europe, which has been ongoing for twenty years, there's not much of a health difference between either of these diets and one that contains meat.

DIETARY NUTRIENT COMPOSITION

(Sobieski, J.G. et al., *Nutr. Res.* 36, 464–477, 2016)

	Meat	Vegetarian	Vegan	WFPB*
Total Fat	30.9	30.0	30.4	~10
Total Sugar	22.9	22.9	22.6	~10

*Approximate goal for WFPB with minimal or no added fat

While vegans consume less animal-based protein, this health advantage is largely compromised by their use of added oils (mostly omega-6 oils, which are pro-inflammatory) and sugar. And about 90% of vegetarians still include a lot of dairy in their diet, which still replaces potentially advantageous plant-based protein with animal-based protein. Unlike plant-based protein, dairy does not have any complex carbohydrates (dietary fiber), antioxidants, and vitamins.

So if your vegan or vegetarian friends and family are feeling unhealthy and thinking they need to return to an animal-based diet, please have them look carefully at what they are eating—switching to a WFPB diet will allow them to achieve the optimal health they're looking for.

The Great Exchange

SUBSTITUTIONS TO CREATE HEALTHY PLANT-BASED RECIPES

OCCASIONALLY, YOU MAY WANT TO CHANGE A FAVORITE animal food–based recipe to a plant-based one (as well as extra-sugary recipes to ones with less-refined sugar). To help, I have put together a list of possible food substitutions. You may also know of others that work well. Use whatever makes the dish tasty for you and your companions. Be creative and experiment!

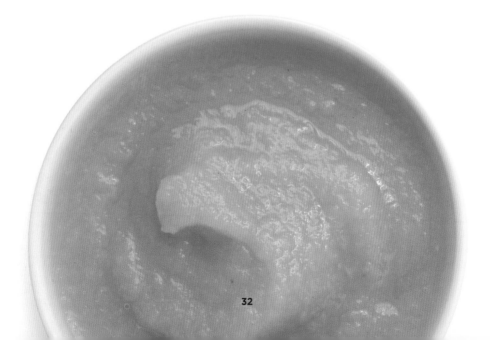

MEAT, POULTRY, OR FISH

Depending on the recipe and your food preferences, you can use your favorite vegetables, beans, grains, or portobello mushrooms, to replace these items. Another food you can use as a substitute while transitioning to a whole foods, plant-based diet is tofu, made from soybeans. Tofu is available in varying consistencies, from very soft (for dressings) to extra-firm (for slicing and crumbling). There is also seitan, a wheat product that comes in plain and spicy flavors, as well as soy hot dogs, veggie burgers, tempeh (made from soybeans), and soy crumbles (similar to ground beef).

WHOLE GRAIN FLOURS

There is a wide variety of whole grain flours, parts of grain flours (endosperm, bran, cracked), and combinations of grain flours (five-grain, seven-grain, nine-grain) on the market. Wheat, oat, triticale, rye, barley, flax, spelt, brown rice, and durum grain flours are just a few examples. When selecting a flour, choose whole grain, not refined.

For some people, their choice of which whole grain flour to use will depend on their sensitivity to gluten, which is found in wheat, barley, and rye. To some extent, determining which grain flour to use in order to avoid this sensitivity is a matter of trial and error.

FATS AND OILS IN MAIN DISHES AND SALADS

When sautéing or frying, use vegetable broth, water, or wine instead of oil. Or simply bake instead of frying. Try preparing dressings with a base of vegetable broth, water, or vinegar rather than the conventional oil.

FATS AND OILS IN CAKES, COOKIES, AND SWEET BREADS

Prune paste is one of the best substitutes for fats and oils in baking; it does not change the taste of the dish as much as other substitutions do. To make prune paste, puree 1 cup of pitted prunes in a food processor with ½ cup of water. To use, substitute one-third the amount of prune paste for the amount of oil called for in the recipe (that is, use ⅓ cup of prune paste to replace 1 cup of oil).

Pureed bananas also work well in some recipes, but they do not hold moisture as successfully as prune paste, and they distort the flavor.

MILK

Nondairy milks include soy, rice, almond, hemp, cashew, coconut, hazelnut, and many others. Experiment with a few different kinds to find one that works best in your recipe. Generally, soy, almond, and coconut milk will produce a thicker product and rice milk a thinner one. When making a creamy sauce or a pudding, I have found the former to be the best replacements.

EGG REPLACERS

There are many different substitutes you can use for eggs. In most cases, you can use whatever is easiest or most convenient for you without affecting taste or consistency. Some examples of substitutes for one egg:

1 tablespoon ground flaxseed mixed with 3 tablespoons water

1 tablespoon chia seed meal mixed with 3 tablespoons water

½ banana, mashed

¼ to ⅓ cup silken tofu

Commercial egg replacer used according to the directions on the box

¼ cup applesauce

Note that, in this cookbook, when an egg substitute is called for in the ingredient list, I use the term "egg replacer."

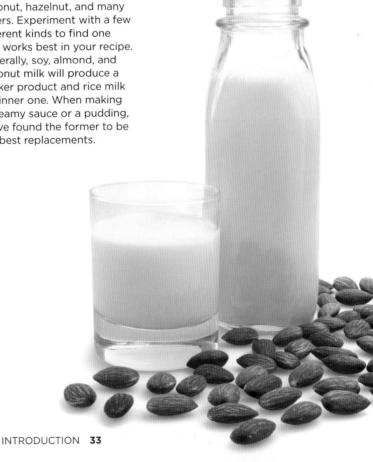

SWEETENERS

When substituting for refined sugar in recipes, try concentrated pure fruit juice—especially apple juice—maple syrup, mashed banana, or any of a wide variety of pureed fruits, including applesauce, preserves, and jams. Dried fruits, such as dates and raisins, work well for baking. Shredded coconut adds a sweet touch, too.

There are basically two categories of sweeteners: wet and dry. Here are a few examples of good substitutions for each:

Wet: brown rice syrup, agave nectar, maple syrup, molasses, fruit syrup, barley malt syrup

Dry: date sugar, stevia, raw sugar, turbinado sugar, Sucanat, evaporated cane juice

The sweetness of each sweetener varies, so you may need to adjust the amount needed to substitute according to taste. I recommend tasting your recipe along the way to determine if more or less is needed.

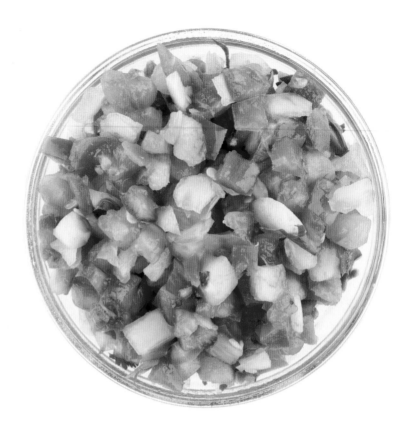

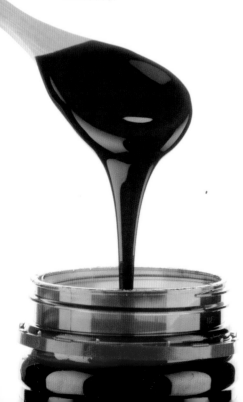

SALT

Depending on the recipe, seasonings such as onion, garlic, parsley, coriander, and celery seed can be used in salt's place. Fresh onion, garlic, lemon juice, salsa, or any type of hot sauce can add zing without sodium (just be careful to check the ingredient list on hot sauces and salsas; some are high in sodium). Low-sodium soy sauce is also delicious in many recipes.

BRANDS WE LIKE

Vegit: An all-purpose seasoning that can be used instead of bouillon to make broth, as a seasoning for soups, and anywhere you would add dried herbs or spices.

Ener-G Egg Replacer: A common commercial egg replacer that works really well. You should use 1½ teaspoons of powdered Ener-G Egg Replacer and 2 tablespoons of water for each egg you're replacing in a recipe.

Mori-Nu: This is a great brand of silken tofu. You can find it in most natural food stores or the health-food aisle of your grocery store. It is shelf-stable, so it won't be in the refrigerated section with the regular tofu.

EVERY CHEF'S TOOLS

EVERY COOK HAS HIS OR HER OWN FAVORITE KITCHEN tools. Here are some that I use on a regular basis:

Sharp knife and cutting board: Everyone has his or her favorite types, but this pair is a must-have in any plant-based kitchen. The great thing about eating a plant-based diet is that you don't need to worry about which cutting board you are using for which foods because there is no fear of cross contamination!

Vegetable peeler: In addition to its regular use, the vegetable peeler is also a great tool to use to julienne vegetables for salads and other dishes.

Slow cooker or pressure cooker: Anyone familiar with these appliances will agree: they save time! They're also a simple and easy way to make a hands-off meal. Many of the soups and stews in this cookbook can be made in a slow cooker or pressure cooker, though you will have to adjust the cooking time.

Griddle: A pancake griddle isn't essential, but griddles are usually much larger than a regular frying pan, allowing you to make more pancakes at a time. In general, griddles either are electric, so you don't need the stove at all, or sit on top of more than one stove burner.

Food processor: Depending on the types of blades or attachments your processor has, you can use this multiuse kitchen gadget to slice, dice, chop, grate, mix, and blend. A lot of the time, you can achieve the same results without a food processor, but for some recipes, such as hummus or pesto, the food processor really is essential.

Blender: This kitchen staple comes in handy, especially when making smoothies or combining liquid ingredients.

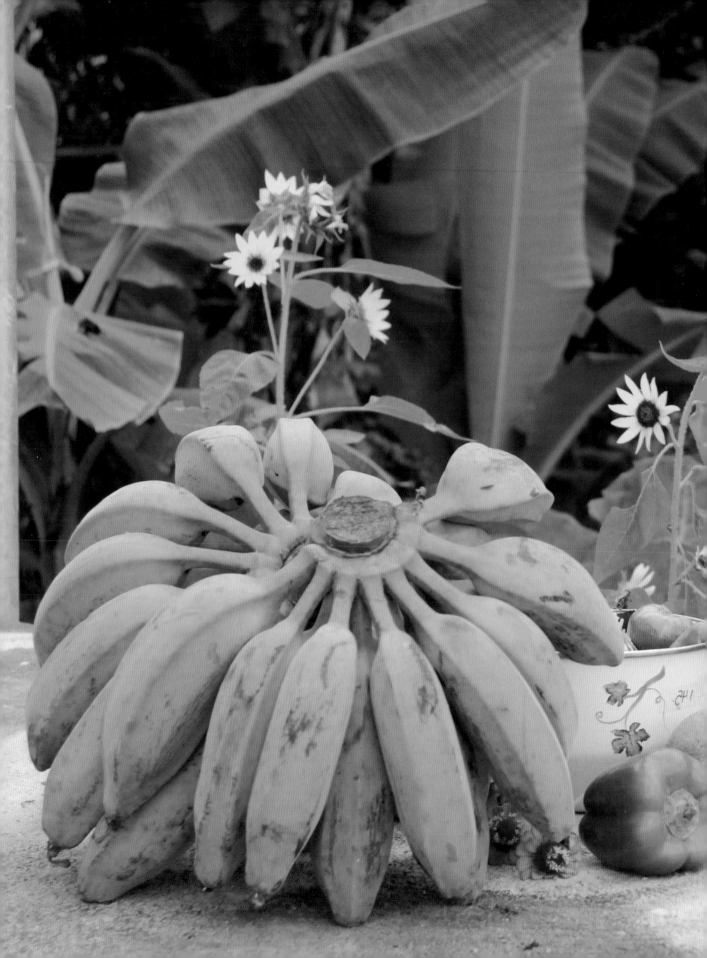

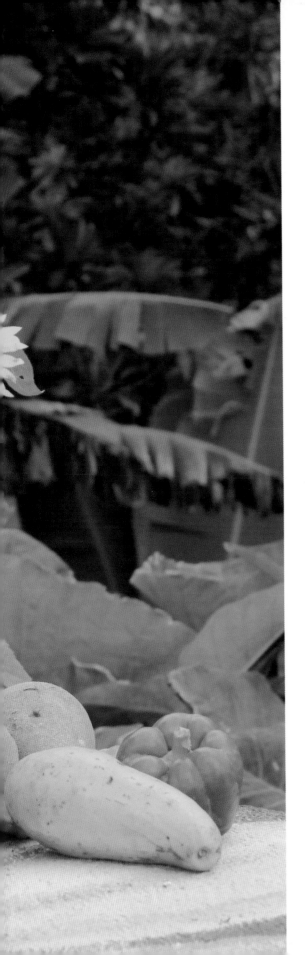

BREADS AND MUFFINS

BANANA WALNUT MUFFINS

MAKES 12 MUFFINS

Bananas in my household never go to waste, even when they are soft and overripe. If I'm not freezing them for my favorite Chocolate Cravings (page 296), I'm using them in this recipe. Taking only 10 minutes to prepare, these muffins are scrumptious with the addition of chopped walnuts.

2 cups whole wheat pastry flour
1 teaspoon baking powder
1 teaspoon baking soda
1 teaspoon ground cinnamon
¼ cup raw cane sugar
¼ cup chopped walnuts
2 ripe bananas
1 cup unsweetened nondairy milk
  (rice, soy, almond, etc.)

Topping
¼ cup raw cane sugar
½ teaspoon ground cinnamon

1. Preheat oven to 350°F.

2. Line a 12-cup muffin tin with paper liners (or use a nonstick pan).

3. Combine flour, baking powder, baking soda, cinnamon, sugar, and walnuts in a medium-size mixing bowl.

4. In a separate bowl, mash bananas and milk together.

5. Fold dry ingredients into wet mixture. Spoon the mixture into the muffin cups.

6. For the topping, mix together sugar and cinnamon in a small bowl. Sprinkle on top of muffins.

7. Bake for 20–25 minutes, until a toothpick inserted into the center of a muffin comes out clean.

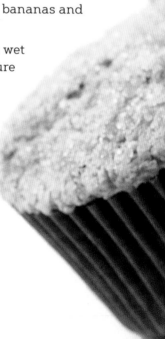

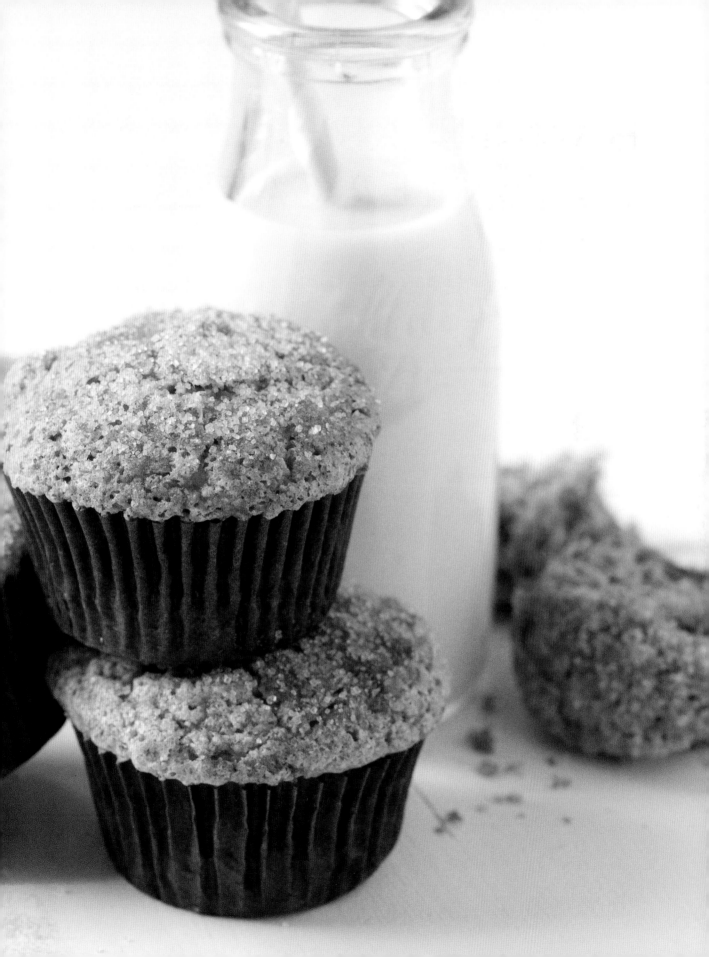

BLACKBERRY LEMON TEA CAKES

MAKES 12 TEA CAKES

Picking blackberries and making pies, cobblers, and lemon tea cakes are fond summertime memories of childhood. This delectable berry is one of our favorite fruits, and it adds a wonderful addition to these tasty lemon tea cakes.

2 cups whole wheat pastry flour

½ cup raw cane sugar

1½ teaspoons baking powder

1½ teaspoons grated lemon zest

1¼ cups unsweetened nondairy milk (rice, soy, almond, etc.)

1 tablespoon lemon juice

1 cup blackberries

2 tablespoons unsweetened shredded coconut

1. Preheat oven to 350°F. Line a baking sheet with parchment.

2. Combine flour, sugar, baking powder, and zest in a medium-size mixing bowl.

3. In a separate bowl, mix together milk and lemon juice.

4. Fold dry ingredients into wet mixture, then gently add the blackberries. Do not overmix.

5. Place 1–2 tablespoons of mixture on lined baking sheet, repeating until mixture is gone. Top with coconut.

6. Bake for 20–25 minutes, until a toothpick inserted into the center of a tea cake comes out clean.

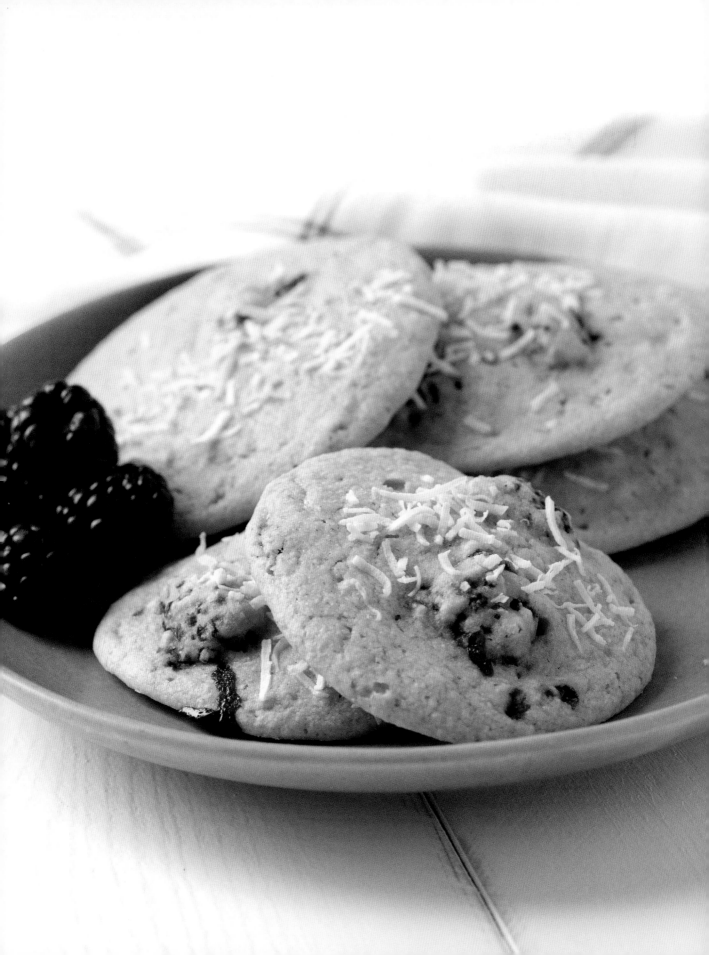

PUMPKIN PIE MUFFINS WITH PECANS

MAKES 12 MUFFINS

On the go, after school, or on the way to soccer practice, you'll find that these muffins make a great snack. And what's better, they take only about 10 minutes to prepare and 20–25 minutes to bake.

2 cups whole wheat pastry flour
½ cup raw cane sugar
1 teaspoon baking powder
1 teaspoon baking soda
1 teaspoon ground cinnamon
½ teaspoon ground ginger
½ teaspoon ground nutmeg
½ teaspoon ground allspice
¼ teaspoon salt
½ cup pumpkin puree
1 cup water
½ cup applesauce
½ cup whole pecans

1. Preheat oven to 350°F.

2. Line a 12-cup muffin tin with paper liners (or use a nonstick pan).

3. Combine flour, sugar, baking powder, baking soda, cinnamon, ginger, nutmeg, allspice, and salt in a medium-size mixing bowl.

4. In a separate bowl, mix together pumpkin puree, water, and applesauce.

5. Fold dry ingredients into wet mixture. Spoon mixture into muffin cups.

6. Gently press a few pecans onto the top of each muffin.

7. Bake for 20–25 minutes, until a toothpick inserted into the center of a muffin comes out clean.

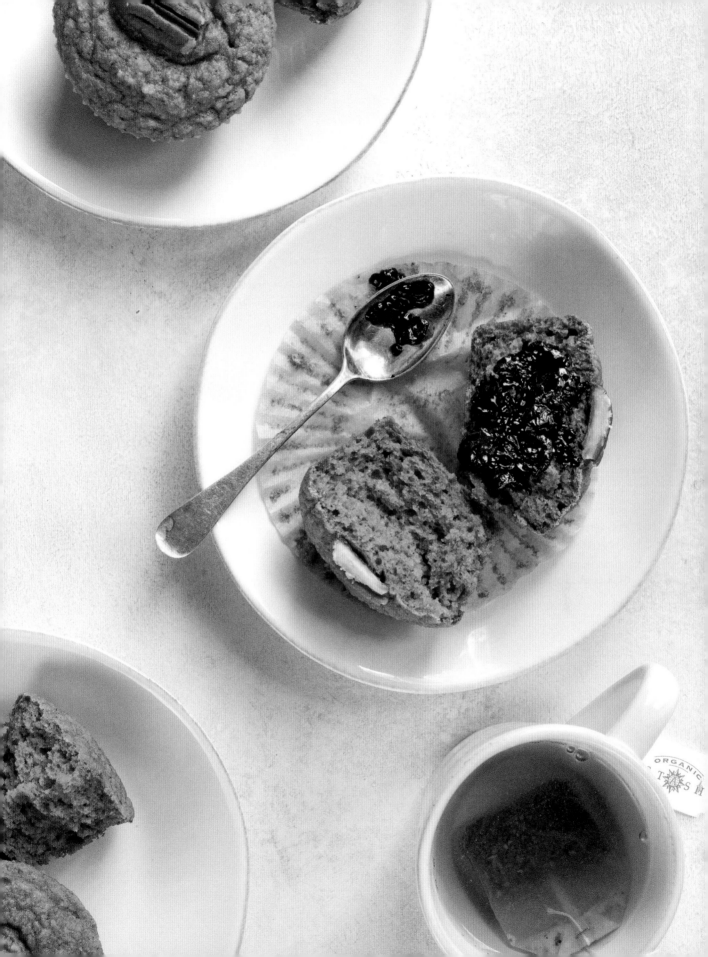

FIESTA CORNBREAD

MAKES 6 SERVINGS

Made with fresh corn kernels, this cornbread is great with hearty stews, beans, and collard greens, such as Quick Three-Bean Soup (page 148), Hearty Salsa Stew (page 140), Fasolia (page 265), and African Vegetables (page 192).

1 cup cornmeal

1 cup whole wheat pastry flour

1 teaspoon baking powder

1 teaspoon baking soda

½ teaspoon sea salt

½ teaspoon dried tarragon

¾ cup corn, fresh off the cob

⅓ cup unsweetened applesauce

2 tablespoons maple syrup

1⅓ cups unsweetened nondairy milk (rice, soy, almond, etc.)

1. Preheat oven to 350°F.

2. Combine cornmeal, flour, baking powder, baking soda, salt, and tarragon in a medium-size mixing bowl.

3. In a separate bowl, mix together corn, applesauce, maple syrup, and milk. Add to the dry ingredients and mix.

4. Pour into 9 × 9-inch nonstick baking dish (or baking dish lined with parchment).

5. Bake for 30–35 minutes, until a toothpick inserted into the center of the cornbread comes out clean.

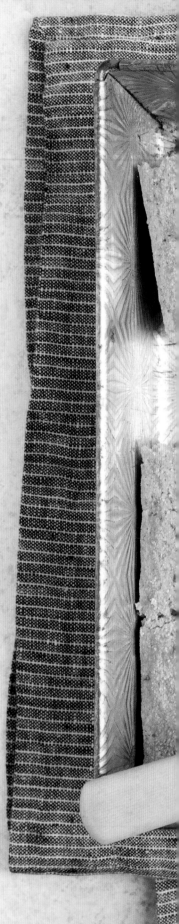

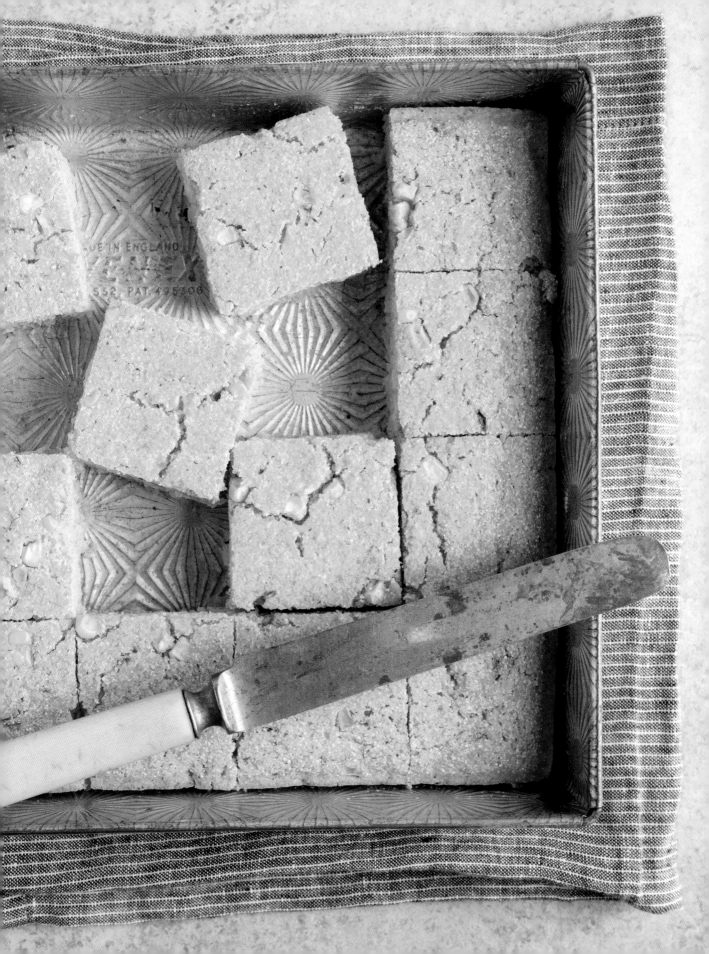

FRUIT BUTTERS

Sweet and creamy, these fruit butters are delicious served on bread, toast, and muffins. Often containing less sugar than jams, they are made by slowly cooking down fresh fruit.

APPLE BUTTER

MAKES 1½ CUPS

10 medium apples, peeled, cored, and roughly chopped
2 tablespoons lemon juice
3 teaspoons ground cinnamon
½ teaspoon ground allspice
¼ cup maple syrup

1. Place all ingredients in a medium-size pot. Cover and cook over low heat, stirring occasionally, for 2 hours, until apples have become thick and all liquid has evaporated.

2. Remove pot from heat and cool, uncovered, for 15 minutes.

3. Transfer mixture to a food processor and pulse until smooth. If there is too much liquid, return to low heat and cook for an additional 15–30 minutes.

note: To make this in a slow cooker, throw all the ingredients together, cook on low for about 6 hours, and blend as instructed.

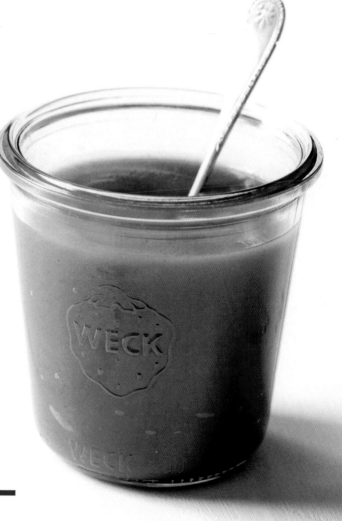

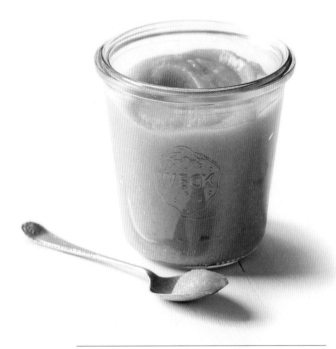

MANGO BUTTER

MAKES 1½ CUPS

2 mangos, peeled and pitted
2 tablespoons maple syrup
2 teaspoons orange juice
2 teaspoons lime juice

1. Scoop mango flesh into a food
    processor and process until
    very smooth.

2. Pour puree into a medium-size
    saucepan. Add maple syrup, orange
    juice, and lime juice.

3. Bring to a bare simmer over medium
    heat and cook, stirring frequently
    and lowering heat if necessary, until
    the mixture is very thick and darkens
    slightly in color, about 1 hour.

4. Let cool. Transfer to an airtight
    container and refrigerate.

PEAR BUTTER

MAKES 1½ CUPS

10 pears, peeled, cored, and diced
1 cup water
3 tablespoons maple syrup
1 tablespoon lemon juice
1 teaspoon ground cinnamon
1 teaspoon ground ginger

1. Place all ingredients in a medium
    saucepan. Cover and cook over
    low heat, stirring occasionally, for
    35–40 minutes, until all liquid has
    evaporated. The mixture should
    be thick.

2. Remove pot from heat and cool,
    uncovered, for 15 minutes.

3. Transfer mixture to a food processor.
    Pulse until smooth.

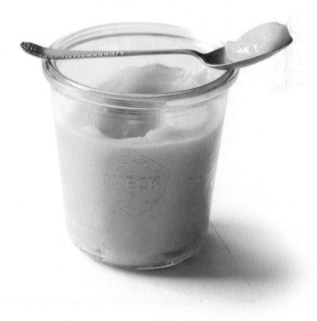

LEMON POPPY MUFFINS

MAKES 12 MUFFINS

Nutty and pleasant-tasting, poppy seeds are a wonderful addition to breads, rolls, bagels, and cakes. And for those who have a sweet tooth, try one of the fruit butters (pages 46–47) with this recipe.

2 cups whole wheat pastry flour

¼ cup poppy seeds

1 teaspoon baking powder

1 teaspoon baking soda

1 teaspoon grated lemon zest

½ cup raw cane sugar

1 cup unsweetened nondairy milk (rice, soy, almond, etc.)

¼ cup lemon juice

1. Preheat oven to 350°F.

2. Line a 12-cup muffin tin with paper liners (or use a nonstick pan).

3. Combine flour, poppy seeds, baking powder, baking soda, lemon zest, and raw cane sugar in a medium-size mixing bowl.

4. In a separate bowl, mix together milk and lemon juice.

5. Fold dry ingredients into wet mixture. Spoon the mixture into the muffin cups.

6. Bake for 20–25 minutes, until a toothpick inserted into the center of a muffin comes out clean.

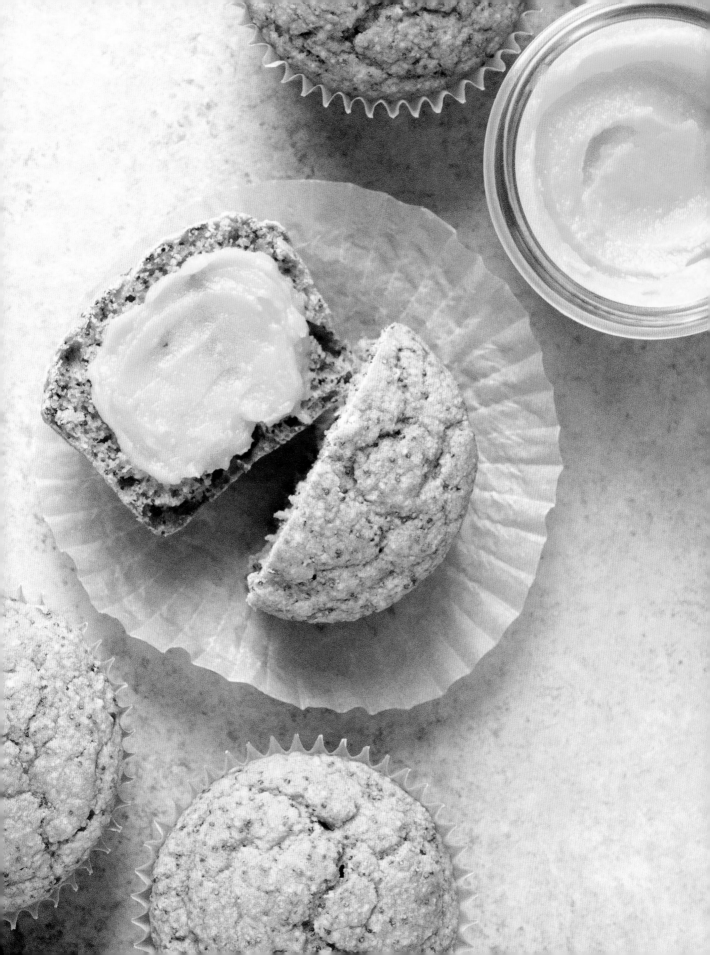

POTATO ROLLS

MAKES 12 ROLLS

My grandmother believed a meal was not complete without bread, and I would blissfully enjoy at least 3 or 4 of her potato rolls. She used oil and dairy, so I've adapted the recipe to make my own tasty and easy version of Granny's famous potato rolls.

2¼ cups whole wheat pastry flour

1 teaspoon salt

2 teaspoons instant (rapid-rise) yeast

1 cup warm unsweetened nondairy milk (rice, soy, almond, etc.)

1½ tablespoons maple syrup

6 tablespoons cooked mashed potatoes

1. In a large bowl, combine flour and salt. Set aside.

2. In a separate bowl, mix together yeast, milk, and maple syrup. Set aside for 5–10 minutes, until a light foam forms.

3. Make a well in the center of the flour and pour in the wet mixture and mashed potatoes. Mix together until a soft dough forms. Place dough on the counter and knead for 1–2 minutes.

4. Divide dough into 12 rolls. Place rolls in a 9 × 13-inch nonstick baking pan (touching is fine). Cover and leave in a warm, draft-free place to double, about 1 hour.

5. Preheat oven to 350°F.

6. Uncover and bake for 20–25 minutes, until golden brown.

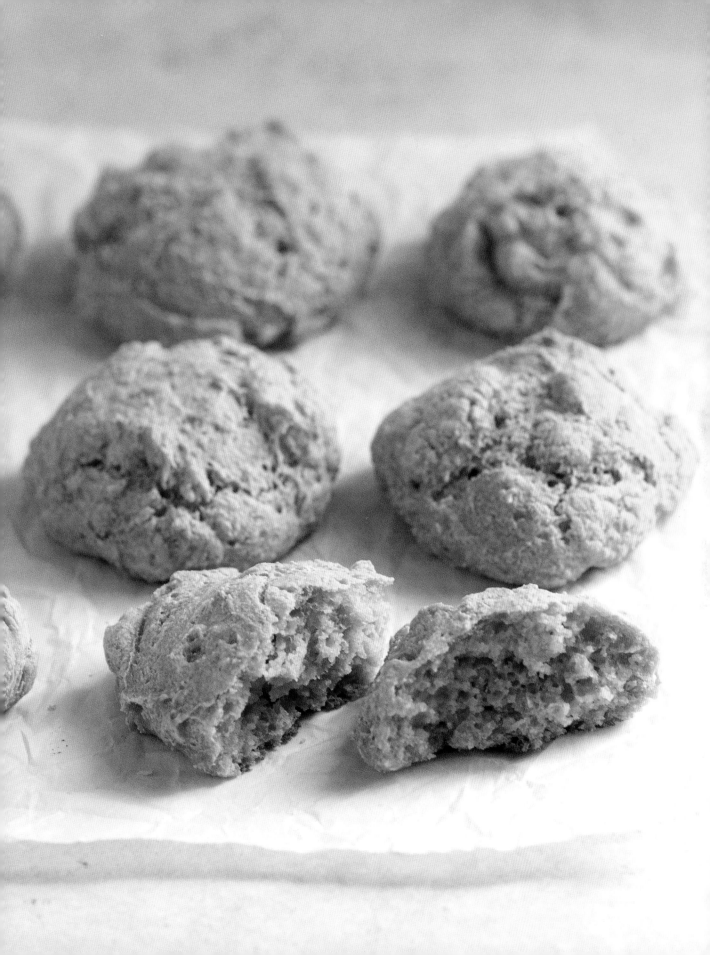

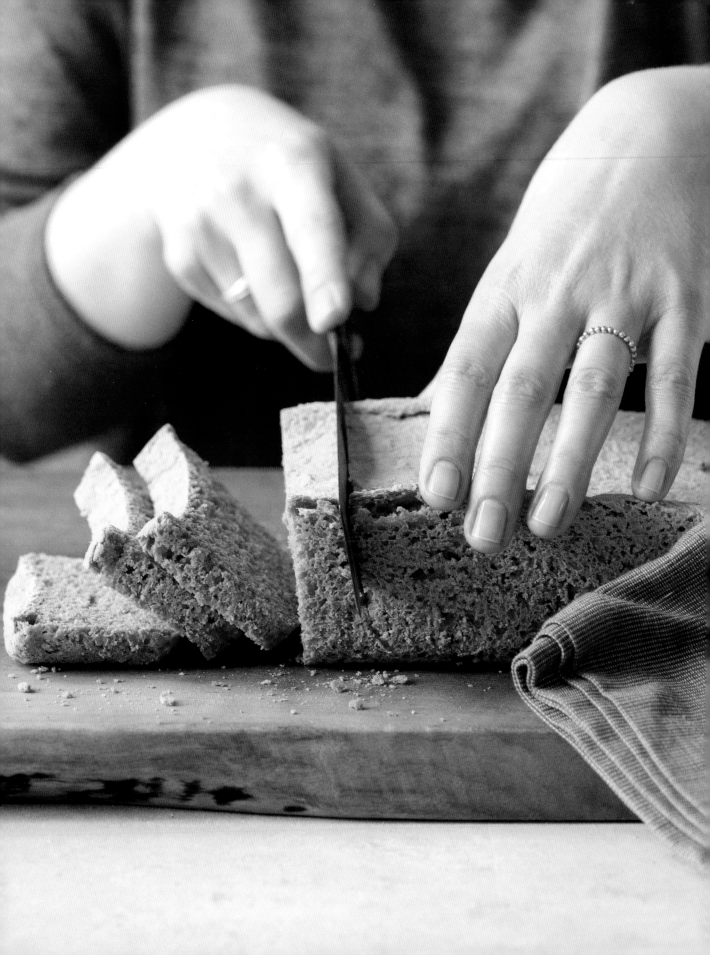

SENSATIONAL HERB BREAD

MAKES 1 LOAF

Once you make this bread, you'll want to make it again and again. Simple and tasty, it goes well with lots of different entrées, as well as soups, salads, and sandwiches. My family loves savory breads, and this is one of our favorites.

2¼ cups whole wheat pastry flour
2 teaspoons onion powder
1½ teaspoons dried oregano
1 teaspoon dried rosemary
1 teaspoon dried basil
½ teaspoon sea salt
2 teaspoons instant (rapid-rise) yeast
1 cup warm water
1 teaspoon molasses

1. In a large bowl, combine flour, onion powder, oregano, rosemary, basil, and salt. Set aside.

2. In a separate bowl, mix together yeast, water, and molasses. Set aside for 5–10 minutes, until a light foam forms.

3. Make a well in the center of the flour and pour in the wet mixture. Mix together until a soft dough forms. Place dough on the counter and knead for 1–2 minutes.

4. Transfer the dough to an 8 × 4-inch nonstick bread pan and cover. Leave in a warm, draft-free place to double, about 1 hour.

5. Preheat oven to 350˚F.

6. Uncover and bake for 30–35 minutes. Bread is done when it sounds hollow when tapped on the top with your knuckles.

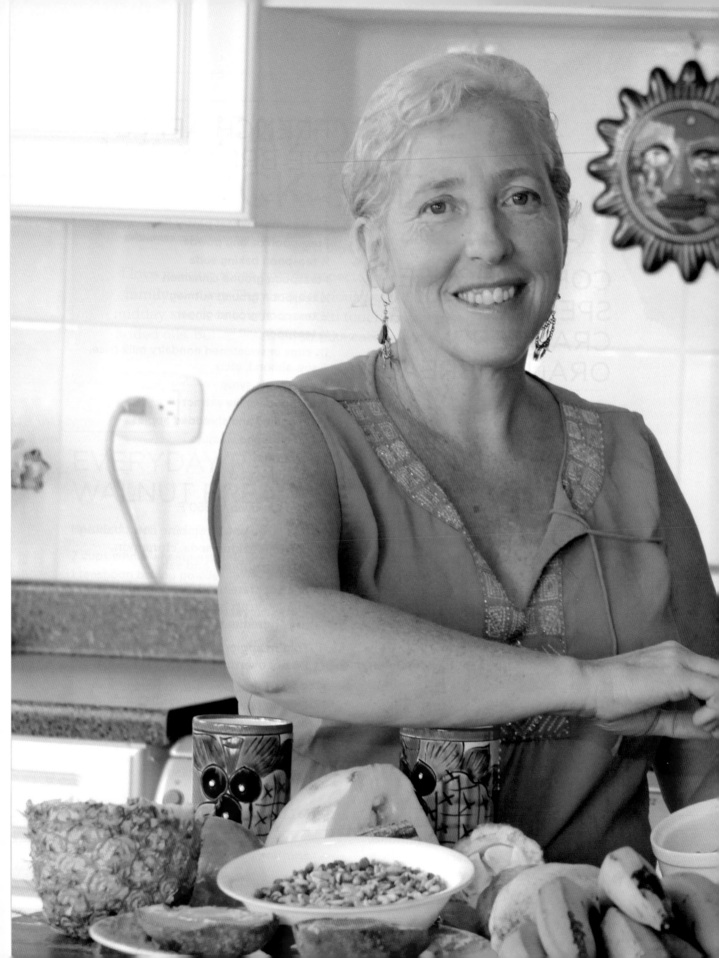

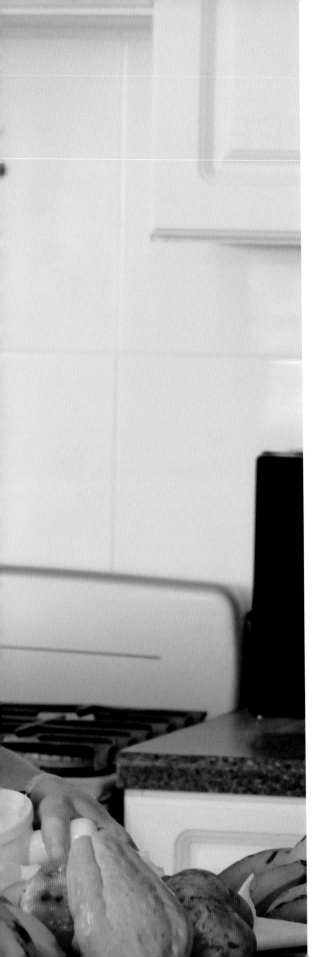

BREAKFAST DISHES

ALMOND-TOPPED BLUEBERRY COFFEE CAKE

MAKES 6 SERVINGS

I was twelve years old when I first made this coffee cake, but at the time, I added a whole stick of butter and cow's milk. By the time I was eighteen, we had transitioned to plant-based milk and had started to decrease the added oils. And guess what, this cake without butter, eggs, and dairy is still one of our favorite morning treats.

2 cups whole wheat pastry flour
1 teaspoon baking powder
½ teaspoon baking soda
1½ teaspoons ground cinnamon
1½ cups unsweetened nondairy milk (rice, soy, almond, etc.)
½ cup maple syrup
½ teaspoon vanilla extract
1 cup blueberries
½ cup walnuts

Topping
3 tablespoons cane sugar
½ teaspoon ground cinnamon
½ cup slivered almonds

1. Preheat oven to 350°F.

2. In a large bowl, combine flour, baking powder, baking soda, and cinnamon.

3. In a separate bowl, mix milk, maple syrup, and vanilla. Add to the flour mixture. Fold in the blueberries and walnuts. Make sure not to overmix.

4. Spread into a 9 × 9-inch nonstick baking pan.

5. In a small bowl, combine sugar, cinnamon, and almonds. Sprinkle over batter.

6. Bake for about 30 minutes, until a toothpick inserted into the center of the cake comes out clean. Cool slightly before serving.

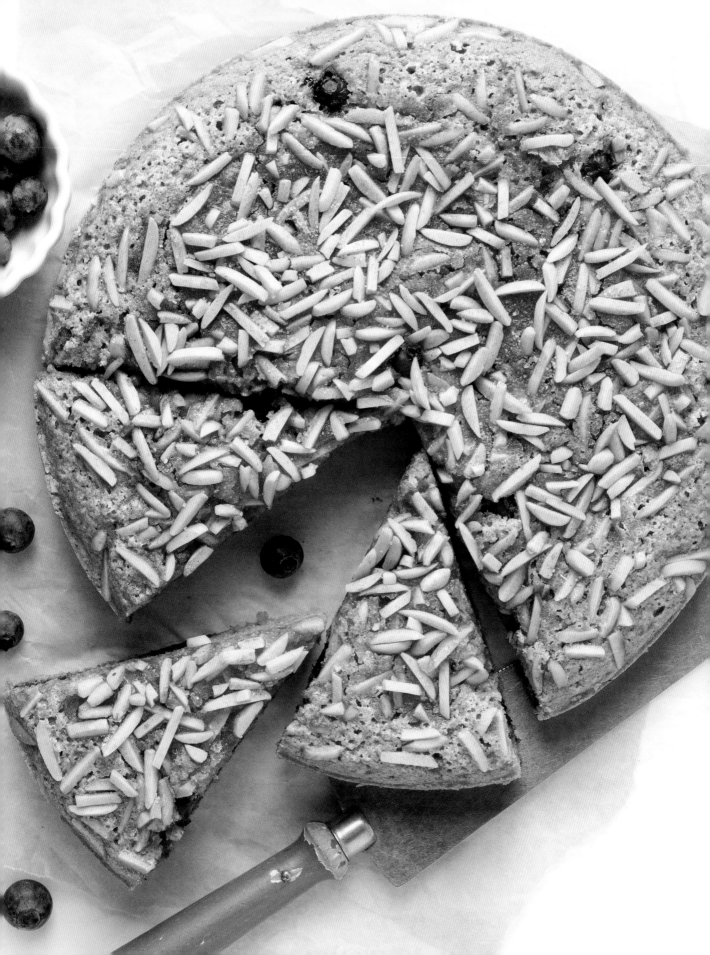

CHIA SEED JAMS

I've always loved homemade jams. Each year my mother and I would go to the local fruit farms and pick buckets of different berries, then make jam, using several cups of white sugar. But just recently, I started making these chia jams and I absolutely love them! They are so simple and can be made quickly with just a fraction of the sugar. And in this case we are not even using white sugar, just maple syrup.

BLACKBERRY GINGER JAM

MAKES 1 CUP

1 cup blackberries
½ teaspoon grated fresh ginger
2 tablespoons maple syrup
1 tablespoon chia seeds

1. In a small saucepan, bring blackberries, ginger, and maple syrup to a simmer over medium-high heat and cook for 4–5 minutes. Mash berries with a fork.

2. Remove jam from heat; taste and add a bit more maple syrup if you prefer a sweeter jam.

3. Return to a boil, then stir in chia seeds; cook for 1 minute to soften seeds. Let jam cool slightly, then transfer to a container. Cover and chill until ready to use.

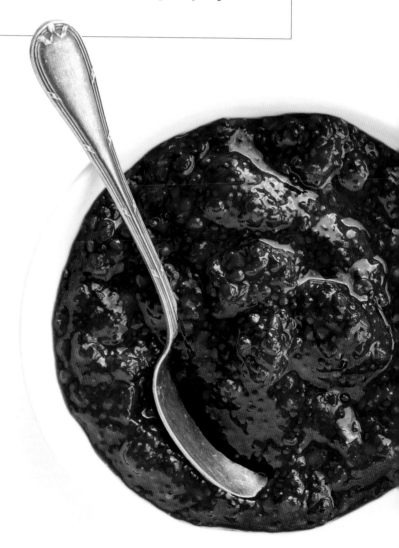

STRAWBERRY ORANGE JAM

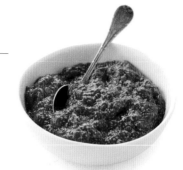

MAKES 1 CUP

1 cup strawberries
1 tablespoon grated orange zest

1 tablespoon maple syrup
1 tablespoon chia seeds

1. In a small saucepan, bring strawberries, orange zest, and maple syrup to a simmer over medium-high heat and cook for 4–5 minutes. Mash berries with a fork.

2. Remove jam from heat; taste and add a bit more maple syrup if you prefer a sweeter jam.

3. Return to a boil, then stir in chia seeds; cook for 1 minute to soften seeds. Let jam cool slightly, then transfer to a container. Cover and chill until ready to use.

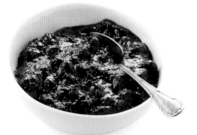

BLUEBERRY MINT JAM

MAKES 1 CUP

1 cup blueberries
2 teaspoons chopped fresh mint

1 tablespoon maple syrup
1 tablespoon chia seeds

1. In a small saucepan, bring blueberries, mint, and maple syrup to a simmer over medium-high heat and cook for 4–5 minutes. Mash berries with a fork.

2. Remove jam from heat; taste and add a bit more maple syrup if you prefer a sweeter jam.

3. Return to a boil, then stir in chia seeds; cook for 1 minute to soften seeds. Let jam cool slightly, then transfer to a container. Cover and chill until ready to use.

PEACH JAM WITH A TOUCH OF CINNAMON

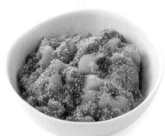

MAKES 1 CUP

1 cup diced peaches
¼ teaspoon ground cinnamon

1 tablespoon maple syrup
1 tablespoon white chia seeds

1. In a small saucepan, bring peaches, cinnamon, and maple syrup to a simmer over medium-high heat and cook for 4–5 minutes.

2. Remove jam from heat; taste and add a bit more maple syrup if you prefer a sweeter jam.

3. Return to a boil and stir in chia seeds; cook for 1 minute to soften seeds. Let jam cool slightly, then transfer to a container. Cover and chill until ready to use.

CHOCOLATE DOMINICANA

MAKES 2 MUGS

This flavorful mug of hot chocolate is a favorite in our SOMOS education center, located in La Cumbre, Dominican Republic. Since we have lots of cacao (chocolate) trees growing in the area, the teachers and students visiting from our US partner schools have this drink once or twice a day, often asking for second and third servings.

2 cups unsweetened nondairy
    milk (rice, soy, almond, etc.)
2 tablespoons rolled oats
1 tablespoon cocoa powder
2 tablespoons cane sugar
1 cinnamon stick
1 teaspoon ground nutmeg
1 teaspoon ground allspice
½ teaspoon ground cloves
Pinch of salt

Add all ingredients to a small pan and bring to a low boil. Cook for 2–3 minutes. Pour into mugs and serve.

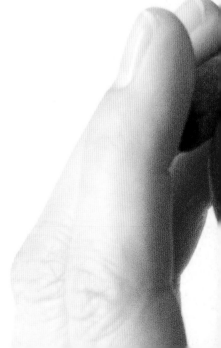

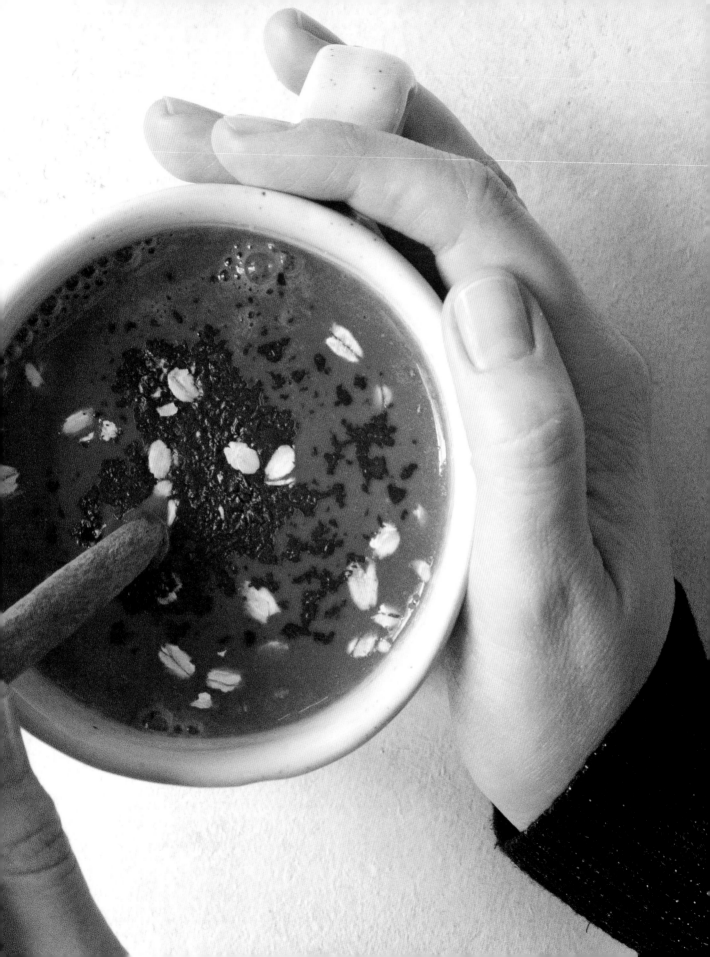

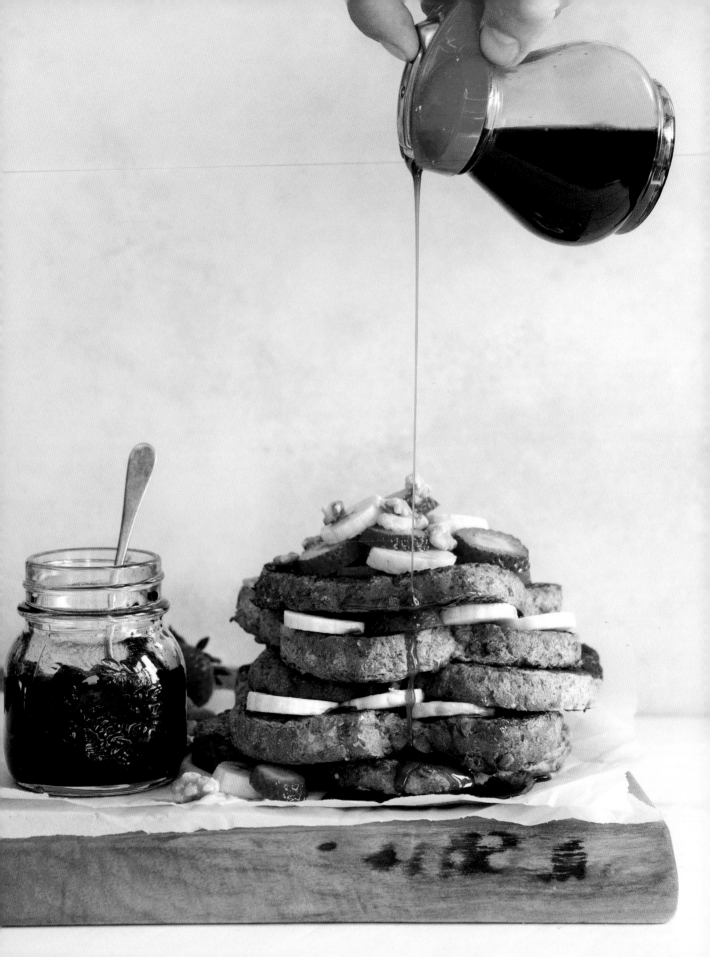

FAVORITE FRENCH TOAST

MAKES 8 SLICES

I love making French toast with leftover quick bread, especially Everyday Raisin Walnut Bread (page 54). Use a good nonstick skillet, and make sure to preheat it.

1 banana, mashed

1 cup unsweetened nondairy milk (soy or almond)

1 tablespoon maple syrup, plus more for serving (optional)

2 tablespoons flaxseed meal (do not mix with water)

1 teaspoon vanilla extract

8 slices whole grain bread

Fresh fruit and/or *Chia Seed Jam* (pages 60–61), for serving

1. Mix banana, milk, maple syrup, flaxseed meal, and vanilla in a large mixing bowl to form batter.

2. Quickly dip both sides of bread into batter.

3. Preheat a nonstick skillet over high heat. Reduce heat to medium-high and cook French toast, in batches, until golden brown on both sides.

4. Serve with fresh fruit, jam, or maple syrup.

FRUIT CRÊPES

MAKES 4-6 CRÊPES

These simple crêpes can be filled with your favorite fruit filling or something savory. When cooking the crêpes, make sure to use a preheated nonstick skillet.

Crêpes

1 cup whole wheat pastry flour

2 egg replacers (2 tablespoons flaxseed meal mixed with 6 tablespoons water)

2 cups unsweetened nondairy milk (rice, soy, almond, etc.)

Filling Suggestions

Sliced berries, banana, or other fresh fruit

Crushed nuts

Chia Seed Jam (pages 60-61)

Fruit Butter (pages 46-47)

Natural peanut butter

Maple syrup

1. In a large bowl, whisk flour, egg replacers, and milk until batter is smooth. Add more milk if needed.

2. Heat a small nonstick skillet over medium heat until hot. Pour about ¼ cup of the batter evenly over bottom of pan. Tilt and rotate the skillet until batter is spread evenly. Cook the crêpe until it is fully cooked. If you try to flip it too soon, it will fold over on itself and stick to the bottom of the skillet. I know it's ready when I shake the pan and it lifts from the side. Once it's ready, flip and cook the other side. Repeat this process with remaining batter.

3. If the batter thickens while you're making the crêpes, thin it with a little extra milk.

4. Serve with your favorite fillings.

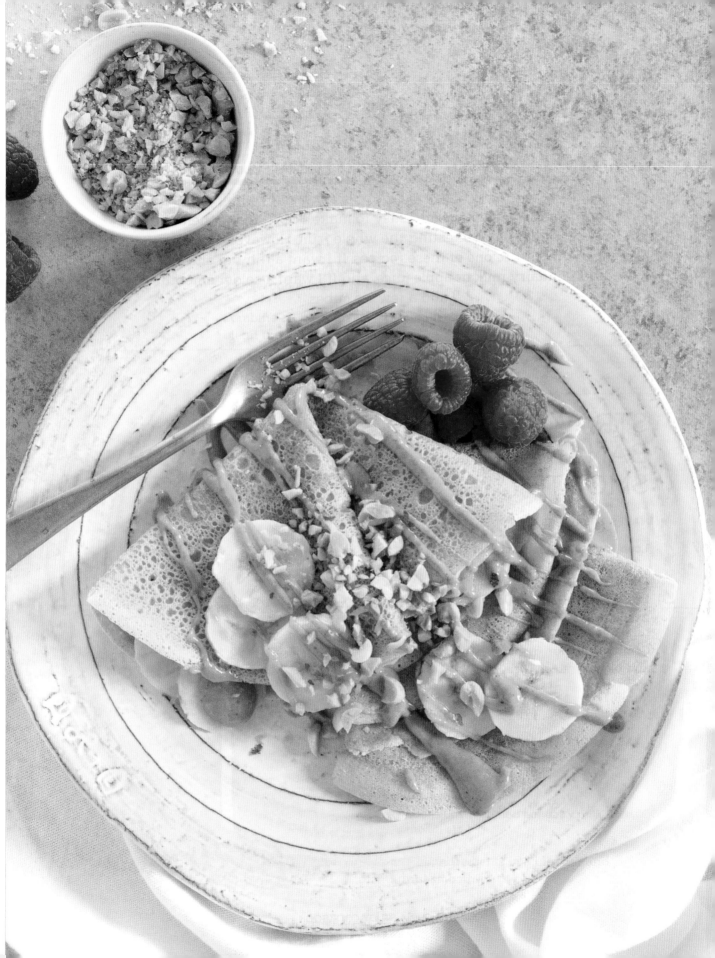

G-MOM'S DAILY FRUIT OATMEAL

MAKES 3 SERVINGS

When asked what I have for breakfast, I often say oatmeal. We love this dish. In terms of fruit, I use whatever is in season. And sometimes I use steel-cut oats in place of old-fashioned oats, then add blackberries, maple syrup, cinnamon, and walnuts, and top it all off with a little nondairy milk. Yummy!

2 cups water
1 cup old-fashioned oats
½ cup raisins
½ cup blueberries
2 teaspoons maple syrup, divided
½ cup sliced strawberries
1–2 kiwis, peeled and diced
Ground cinnamon, to taste
1 teaspoon ground flaxseed, per bowl
Chopped walnuts, for topping (optional)

1. In a small pot, bring water to a boil over medium-high heat. Add oats and raisins and stir until thick, 2–3 minutes.

2. Place blueberries in the bottom of a serving bowl. Drizzle with 1 teaspoon of maple syrup.

3. Pour cooked oatmeal over blueberries. Place strawberries and kiwis on top of oatmeal. Sprinkle cinnamon and flaxseed on top of oatmeal. Drizzle with remaining 1 teaspoon of maple syrup and add walnuts (if using).

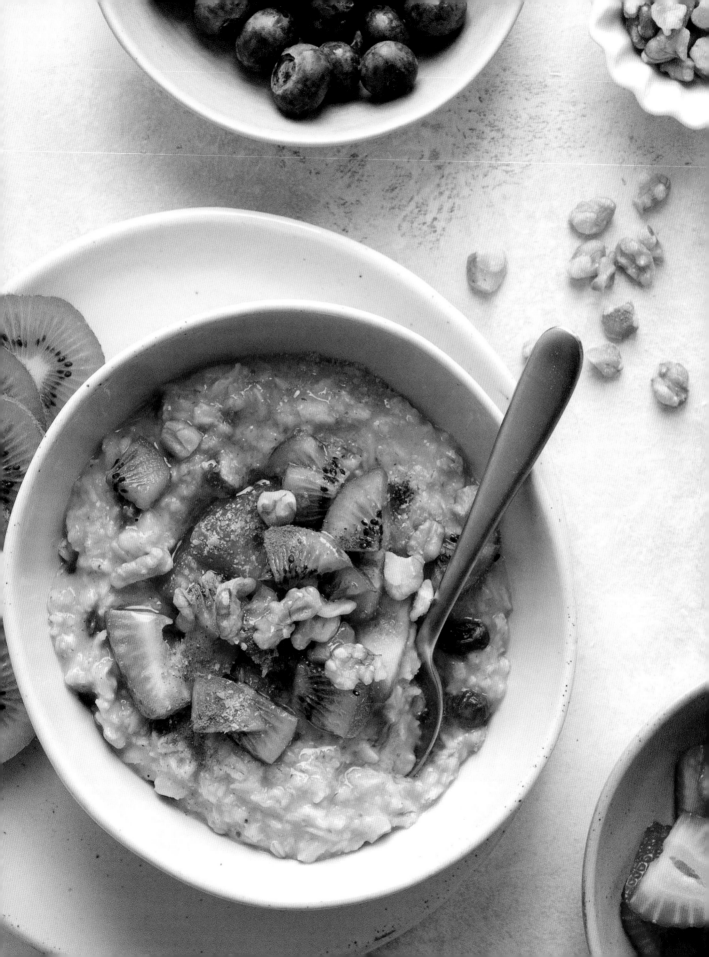

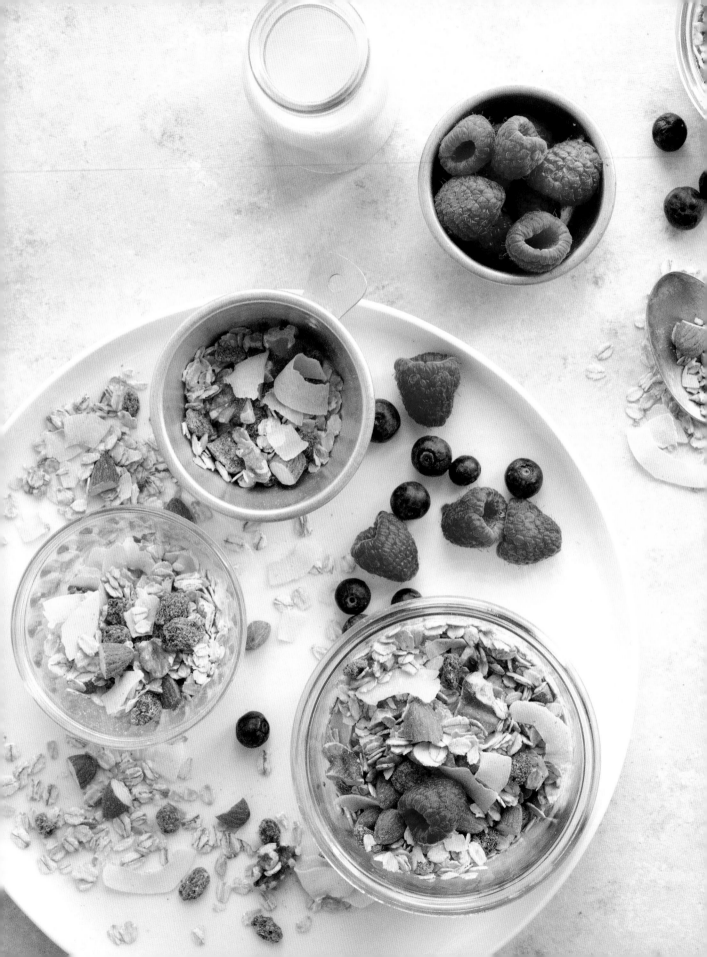

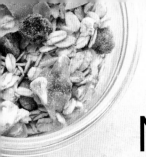

MUESLI

MAKES 7½ CUPS

This versatile and easy breakfast cereal can be served with cold nondairy milk or cooked up like oatmeal. As with any cereal, adding fresh fruit—like peaches, strawberries, or blueberries—makes it even more delicious. And what's nice about this cereal is that it can keep for up to 2 months at room temperature.

4½ cups rolled oats
1 cup raisins
½ cup chopped dried fruit
½ cup chopped walnuts
½ cup chopped almonds
½ cup unsweetened shredded coconut
¼ cup roasted sunflower seeds

1. Combine all ingredients in a large bowl. Mix well.

2. Store in an airtight container.

NATURE'S GRANOLA

MAKES 12 SERVINGS

I love having a large container of this granola available. It's perfect for breakfast and snacks or for topping off Yogurt Parfaits (page 84) and Chocolate Cravings (page 296). This easy recipe is delicious served with just blackberries, strawberries, and your favorite plant-based milk.

1 cup water

½ cup cane sugar

⅓ cup maple syrup

2 teaspoons vanilla extract

4½ cups rolled oats

1 cup unsweetened shredded coconut

1 cup raisins

½ cup chopped dried fruit

½ cup slivered almonds

½ cup chopped pecans

1 teaspoon ground cinnamon

½ teaspoon ground nutmeg

1. Preheat oven to 300°F. Line a baking sheet with parchment.

2. Add water, cane sugar, maple syrup, and vanilla to a large saucepan. Cook over medium heat for 2–3 minutes, until sugar is dissolved.

3. In a large bowl, mix together oats, coconut, raisins, dried fruit, almonds, pecans, cinnamon, and nutmeg. Add wet mixture and mix until coated.

4. Thinly spread mixture on lined baking sheet.

5. Bake, stirring every 15 minutes, for about 1 hour, until golden brown.

6. Let cool and then transfer to an airtight container.

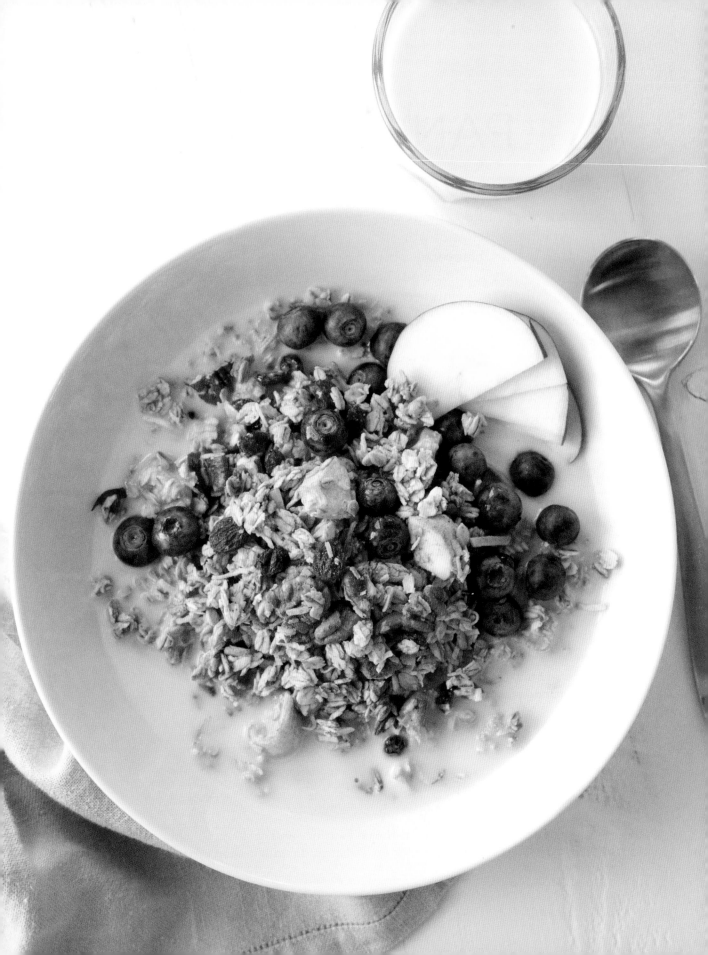

PANCAKES

I have fond childhood memories of Saturday morning pancakes piled high with lots of wonderful fruit syrups: sour cherries, strawberries, blueberries, blackberries, peaches, and even applesauce. My mother would boil 2 cups of berries with ¼ cup of water, then add a mixture of cornstarch (1 tablespoon), water (¼ cup), and a sweetener (1–2 tablespoons). Once the fruit sauce became thick, she would serve it with our pancakes, making it one of our favorite breakfast meals of the week!

PANANA CAKES

MAKES 12 PANCAKES

2 cups whole wheat pastry flour
1 teaspoon baking soda
1 teaspoon baking powder
½ teaspoon sea salt
1½ cups unsweetened nondairy milk (rice, soy, almond, etc.)
⅓ cup applesauce
2 egg replacers (2 tablespoons flaxseed meal mixed with 6 tablespoons water)
1 tablespoon maple syrup

1. In a large bowl, combine flour, baking soda, baking powder, and salt.

2. In a separate bowl, mix milk, applesauce, egg replacers, and maple syrup.

3. Combine the wet and dry ingredients. Stir to remove any lumps. The batter should be pourable; if it seems too thick, add more milk.

4. Preheat a nonstick skillet or griddle.

5. Pour small amounts of batter onto the heated surface and cook until the top bubbles. Turn with a spatula and cook the second side until golden brown. Serve immediately.

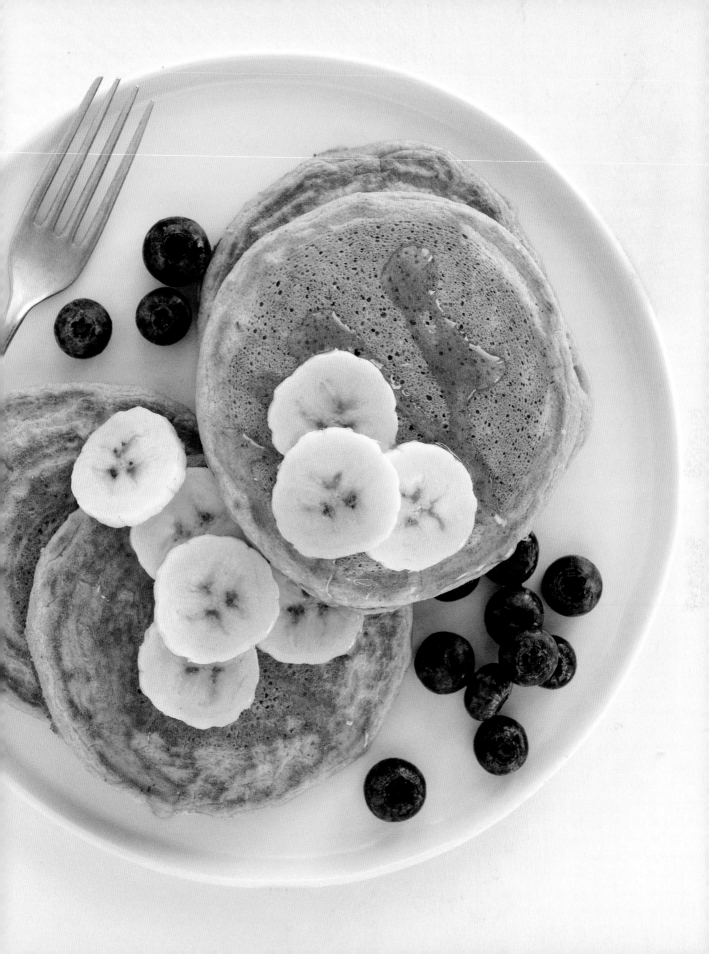

PUMPKIN PANCAKES

MAKES 12 PANCAKES

2 cups whole wheat pastry flour
1 teaspoon baking soda
1 teaspoon baking powder
½ teaspoon sea salt
1 tablespoon pumpkin pie spice
2½ cups unsweetened nondairy milk (rice, soy, almond, etc.)
½ cup pumpkin puree
2 egg replacers (2 tablespoons flaxseed meal mixed with 6 tablespoons water)
2 tablespoons maple syrup

1. In a large bowl, combine flour, baking soda, baking powder, salt, and pumpkin pie spice.

2. In a separate bowl, mix milk, pumpkin puree, egg replacers, and maple syrup.

3. Combine the wet and dry ingredients. Stir to remove any lumps. The batter should be pourable; if it seems too thick, add more milk.

4. Preheat a nonstick skillet or griddle.

5. Pour small amounts of batter onto the heated surface and cook until the top bubbles. Turn with a spatula and cook the second side until golden brown. Serve immediately.

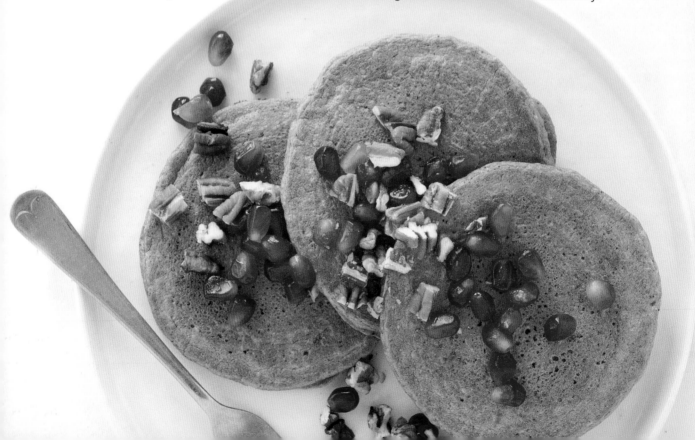

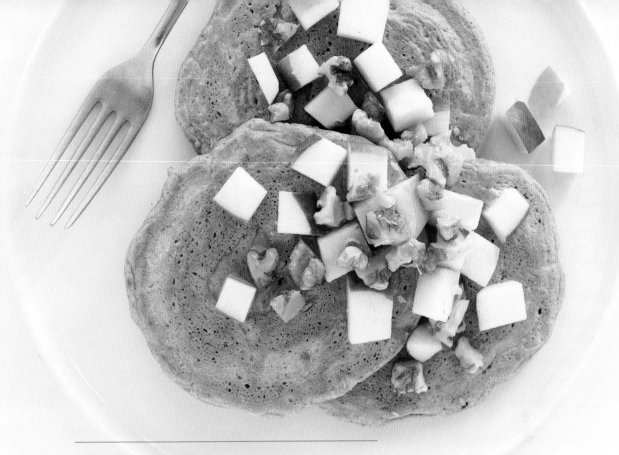

APPLE PIE PANCAKES

MAKES 12 PANCAKES

2 cups whole wheat pastry flour

1 teaspoon baking soda

1 teaspoon baking powder

½ teaspoon sea salt

1½ teaspoons ground cinnamon

1½ cups unsweetened nondairy milk (rice, soy, almond, etc.)

2 egg replacers (2 tablespoons flaxseed meal mixed with 6 tablespoons water)

1 tablespoon maple syrup

1 cup peeled shredded apples

½ cup chopped walnuts

1. In a large bowl, combine flour, baking soda, baking powder, salt, and cinnamon.

2. In a separate bowl, mix milk, egg replacers, and maple syrup.

3. Combine the wet and dry ingredients. Add apples and walnuts. Stir to remove any lumps. The batter should be pourable; if it seems too thick, add more milk.

4. Preheat a nonstick skillet or griddle.

5. Pour small amounts of batter onto the heated surface and cook until the top bubbles. Turn with a spatula and cook the second side until golden brown. Serve immediately.

SAVORY SOUTHWESTERN BURRITOS

MAKES 6–7 BURRITOS

For those who like a more savory, salty breakfast, this burrito is our favorite. And as my sons can attest, these oh-so-good breakfast burritos can be served at any time of the day—breakfast, lunch, or dinner!

4 large potatoes, diced
Onion powder and sea salt,
   to taste
6–7 large whole grain tortillas
1 recipe *Scrambled Tofu* (page 82)
1 (15-ounce) can black beans,
   rinsed and drained
1 (15-ounce) jar salsa

1. Preheat oven to 375˚F.

2. Spread diced potatoes on a nonstick baking sheet. Season with onion powder and salt. After 15 minutes, flip the potatoes, then continue cooking for an additional 15–20 minutes.

3. Place ¼ cup of potatoes in the center of each tortilla, top with ¼ cup of tofu mixture, then add 2 tablespoons of black beans.

4. Fold the bottom of the burrito over, then fold over both sides.

5. Place burritos, seam-side down, in a nonstick baking dish. Spread salsa across top of burritos.

6. Bake for 10 minutes. Serve immediately.

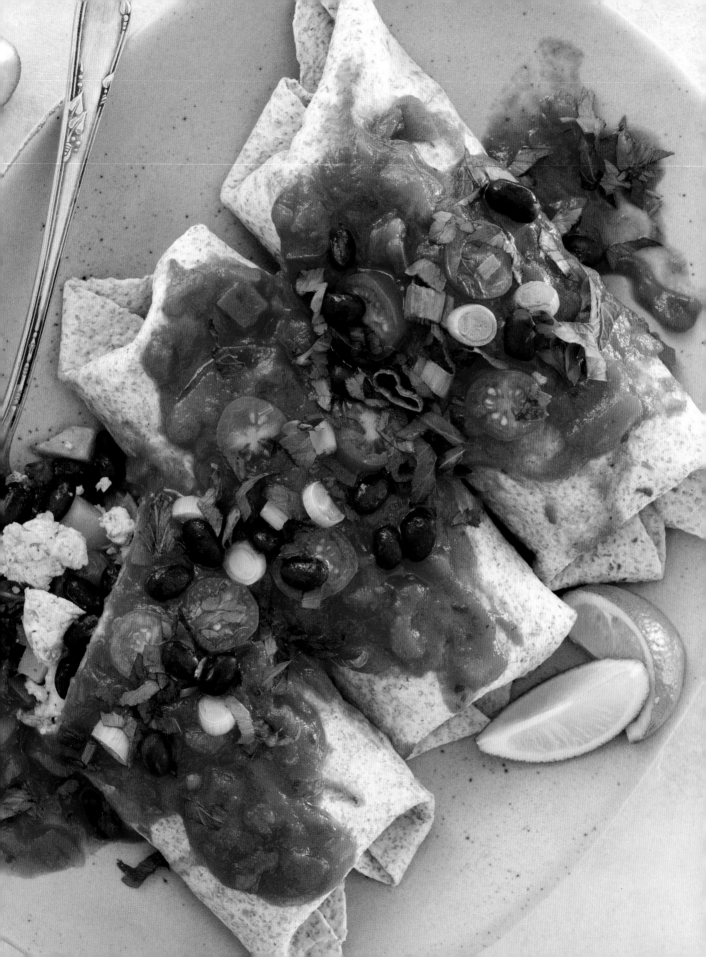

SCRAMBLED TOFU

MAKES 4 SERVINGS

This simple scrambled tofu recipe can be spiced up with additional vegetables. For instance, my younger son likes to add 2–3 handfuls of spinach, kale, or other greens and serves it with diced potatoes, toast, and grits.

½ **large onion, diced**

½ **large carrot, grated**

2 **garlic cloves, minced**

2 **tablespoons vegetable broth**

1 **teaspoon curry powder**

1½ **teaspoons light miso**

1 **(14-ounce) package firm silken tofu, crumbled**

Sea salt and black pepper, to taste

8 **chopped cherry tomatoes (optional)**

¼ **cup finely chopped kale (optional)**

1. In a nonstick pan, gently sauté onion, carrot, and garlic in vegetable broth over medium-high heat until onion browns.

2. Reduce heat to medium and add curry powder. Cook for 1–2 minutes, then add miso and tofu, and cook for an additional 3–4 minutes.

3. Add salt and pepper. If desired, stir in cherry tomatoes and/or kale. Serve warm.

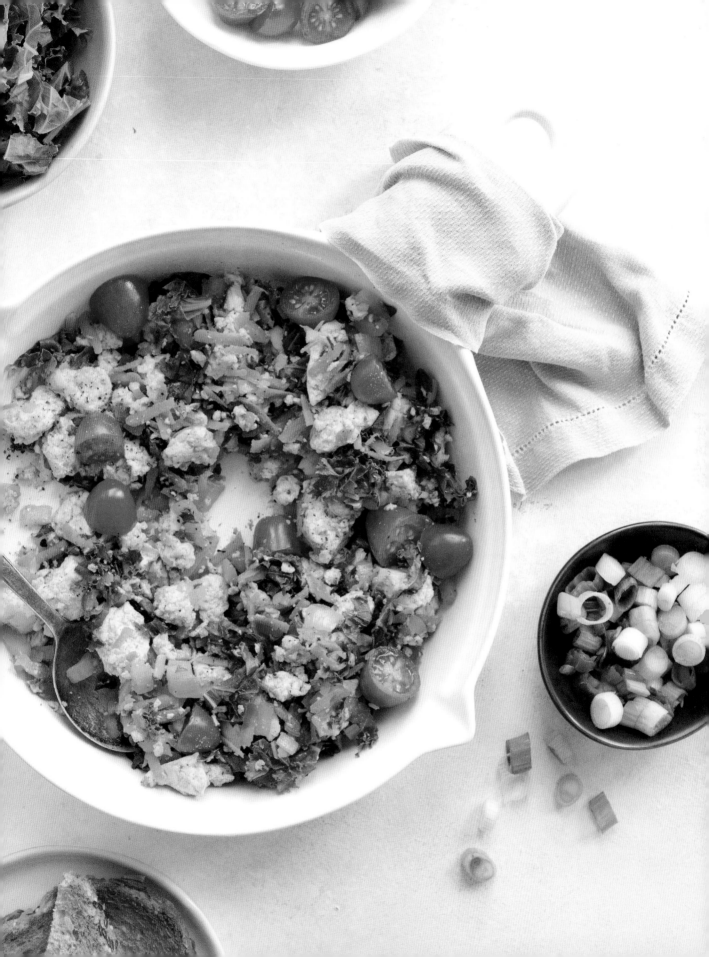

YOGURT PARFAITS

MAKES 1 SERVING

I recently bought an Instant Pot and have found that making yogurt is super easy. With homemade yogurt on hand, I can now make these simple parfaits whenever I want. I like to use my Nature's Granola (page 74) recipe and a lot of fresh fruit.

6 tablespoons *Nature's Granola* (page 74)

1 cup sliced fresh fruit (strawberries, blueberries, raspberries, blackberries, pomegranates, mangos, etc.)

¾ cup soy yogurt or *Instant Pot Yogurt* (below)

Maple syrup

1. Place half of the granola in the bottom of a parfait glass. Top with half of the fresh fruit.

2. Add half of the yogurt. Drizzle with a bit of maple syrup. Repeat layers. Serve immediately.

INSTANT POT YOGURT

1 quart plain organic soy milk, at room temperature (I have found WestSoy to be the best.)

5 Solgar Advanced 40 Plus Acidophilus Vegetable Capsules

1. First, make sure the glass canning jars fit into the bottom of your instant pot.

2. Clean jars with soap and hot water. Dry and set aside.

3. Pour soy milk into a blender. Open capsules and pour powder into the blender. Throw away outer shells of capsules.

4. Blend on high for 3–4 minutes, until powder is evenly mixed throughout milk.

5. Pour mixture into 5 clean, dry jars, making sure to leave ½–¾ inch air space at the top. Place lids on jars and then place in the Instant Pot. Cover, push the "yogurt" button, and set for 12 hours. (It generally sets in 8 hours, but it tastes more like yogurt if you let it process longer.)

6. When done, refrigerate for 5–6 hours before using.

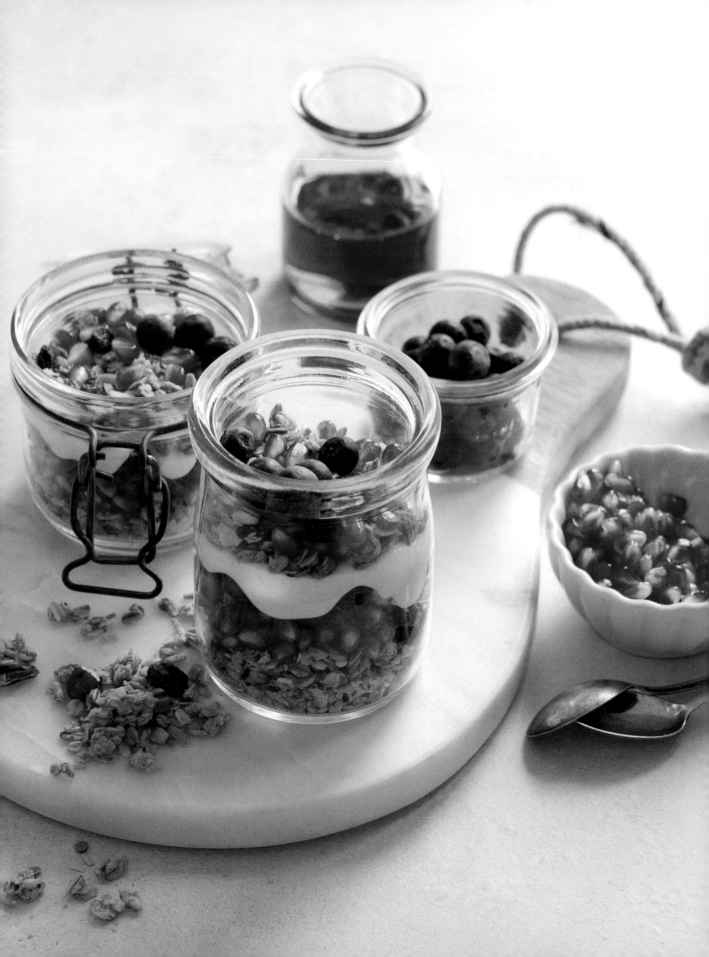

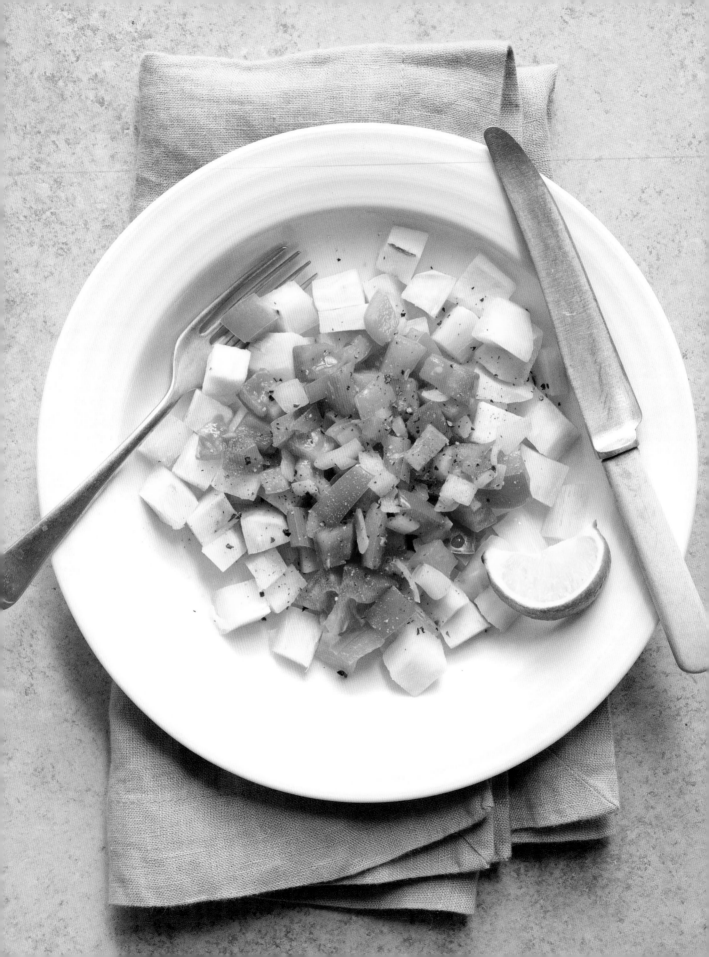

CASSAVA (YUCA) CON CEBOLLAS

MAKES 2–3 SERVINGS

From an early age, this easy, tasty dish was my younger son's favorite Dominican Garden recipe. Our favorite among the root crops is yuca (also known as cassava), which can be purchased in most supermarkets. It can be replaced with any potato or sweet potato, batata, breadfruit, plantain, or banana.

4 cups chopped cassava

1 cup water

1 teaspoon salt, plus more to taste

½ cup chopped onions

½ cup diced tomatoes

¼ cup diced green bell peppers

2 teaspoons lime juice

1. Peel cassava, then cut down the middle lengthwise. Place cassava face down on the cutting board and slice lengthwise one more time. Cut out the stiff fiber in the middle of the cassava, then chop into 1-inch cubes. You should have about 4 cups.

2. Place cassava in a pot and add water and salt. Cover and bring to a simmer over medium heat, then cook for about 30 minutes, until soft. Cooking time depends on the age of the cassava. Check every 2 minutes to see if it's soft, like a potato. When cooked, drain the liquid and set cassava aside.

3. In a skillet, combine onions, tomatoes, bell peppers, and lime juice and cook over medium-high heat for 1–2 minutes, until slightly soft. Do not overcook. Season with salt, then remove from the heat.

4. Place cassava on a serving plate and top with cooked vegetables. Serve warm.

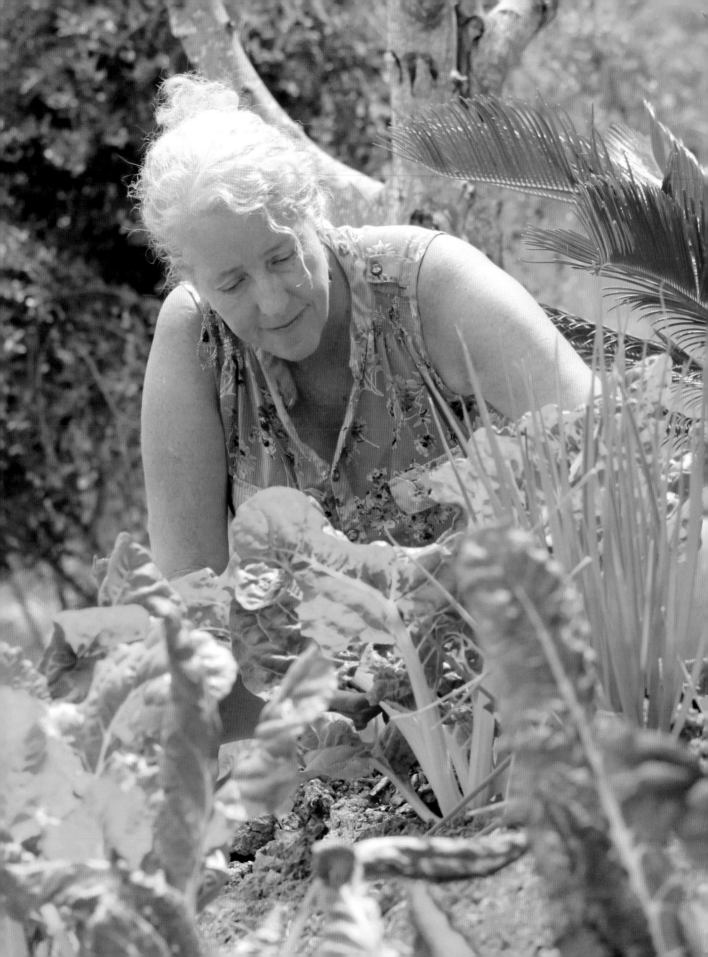

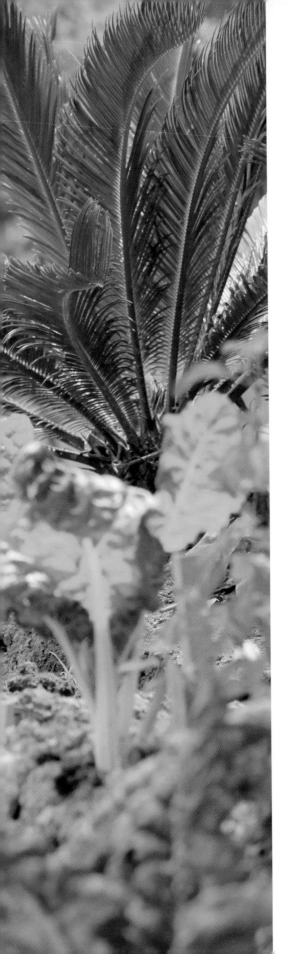

APPETIZERS AND SALADS

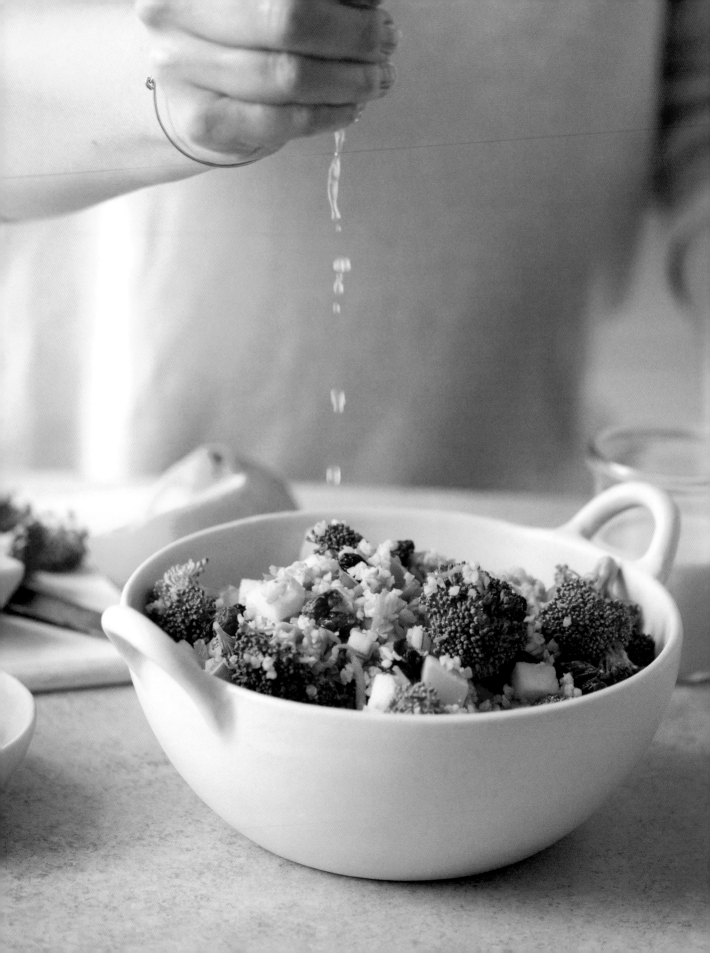

APPLE LEMON BULGUR SALAD

MAKES 5-6 SERVINGS

This simple salad can be made with many different grains. My favorite is bulgur, but if I don't have it on hand, I substitute brown rice. And if I need to replace the vegetables, I try to use crunchy vegetables, such as cauliflower or bell peppers.

2½ cups cooked bulgur

1 cup chopped broccoli

1 cup grated carrots

1 cup chopped apples or pears

½ cup raisins

¼ cup finely diced red onion

½ cup *Lemon Tahini Dressing* (page 103)

Combine all ingredients in a large bowl and toss to mix.

ASIAN GINGER CABBAGE SALAD

MAKES 5½ CUPS

This recipe is a take on classic papaya salad. Green papayas are generally hard to find, so, I've replaced them with shredded cabbage. It's still one of my favorite salads! The gingery dressing, peanuts, and limes go well with the cabbage, green beans, and green onions.

4 cups grated cabbage

1 cup green beans, sliced lengthwise

¼ cup chopped green onions

¼ cup chopped fresh cilantro

½ cup *Asian Ginger Dressing* (page 103)

½ cup crushed peanuts

1 cup *Baked Tofu Cubes* (page 95) (optional)

Lime wedges, for serving

1. Combine cabbage, green beans, green onions, and cilantro in a salad bowl.

2. Fold in the dressing. Top with crushed peanuts and tofu cubes (if using). Serve with lime wedges.

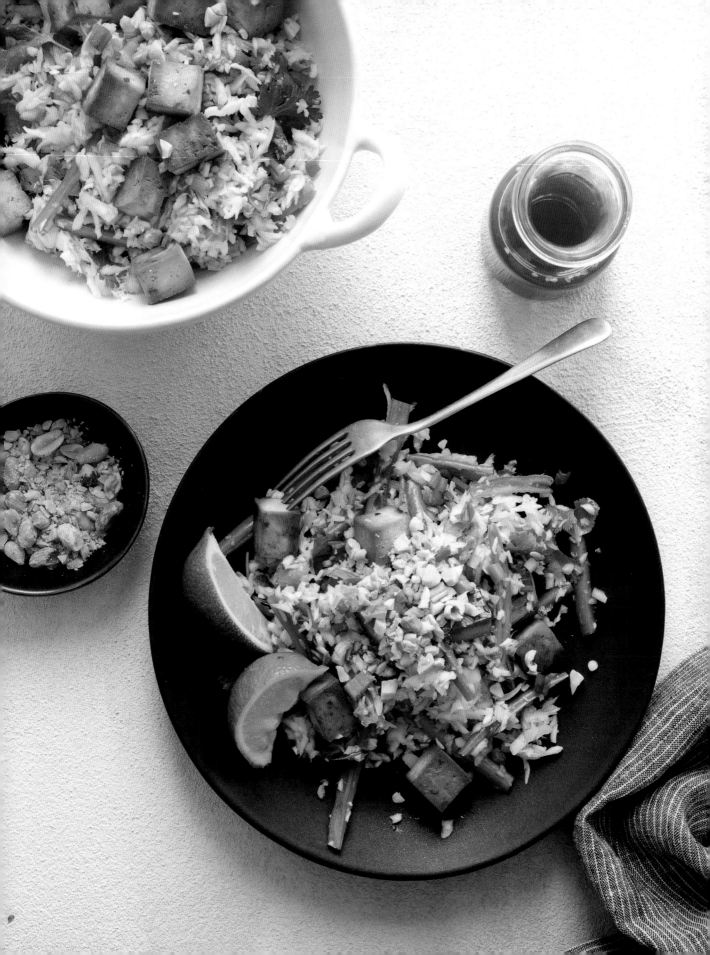

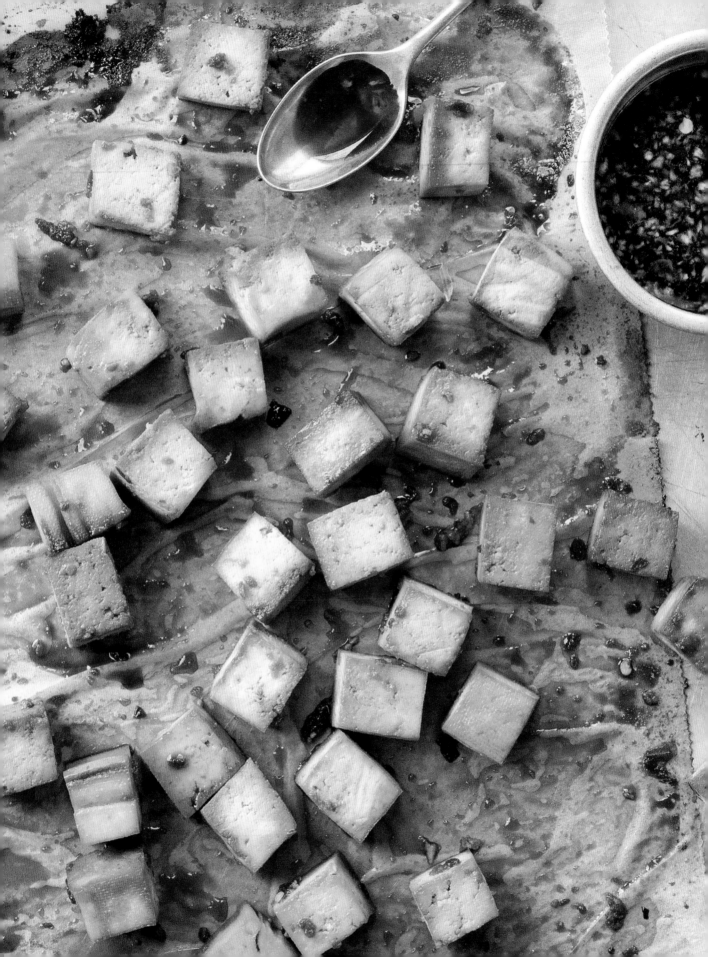

BAKED TOFU CUBES

MAKES 4 SERVINGS

Just recently, I started making my own tofu, using organic soy beans that grow in the Dominican Republic Global Roots center. First, I make soy milk, then boil the milk, add a bit of vinegar, bring it to a curdle, strain it, and voilà—I have the beginnings of tofu. These tofu cubes can be eaten on their own, but they also make a great addition to salads, wraps, and even soups.

3 tablespoons soy sauce
2 tablespoons maple syrup
1 tablespoon rice vinegar
1 teaspoon minced garlic
⅛ teaspoon red pepper flakes
1 (14-ounce) package extra-firm
   tofu, cut into 1-inch cubes

1. Preheat oven to 350°F and line a baking sheet with parchment.

2. In a shallow dish, whisk together soy sauce, maple syrup, rice vinegar, garlic, and red pepper flakes.

3. Coat each piece of tofu in the sauce, then lay flat on lined baking sheet. Drizzle remaining sauce on tofu.

4. Cover with aluminum foil and bake for 15 minutes, then flip each piece of tofu and bake, uncovered, for 20 minutes more.

BROCCOLI WALNUT SALAD

MAKES 6 SERVINGS

A perfect complement to any meal, this crunchy salad is traditionally prepared with bacon and cheddar cheese. In place of these items, I've used walnuts and Golden Garden Mayonnaise (page 184). It's a great salad to take to potlucks and holds up well the next day.

4 cups broccoli florets

½ cup dried cranberries

¼ cup chopped red onion

½ cup chopped walnuts

1–2 tablespoons raw cane sugar

3 tablespoons rice vinegar

¾ cup *Golden Garden Mayonnaise* (page 184)

Salt, to taste

1. In salad bowl, add broccoli, dried cranberries, red onion, and walnuts.

2. In separate bowl, mix 1 tablespoon sugar, rice vinegar, and mayonnaise. Taste and, if needed, add 1 additional tablespoon sugar.

3. Add dressing mixture to broccoli and toss to mix. Season with salt.

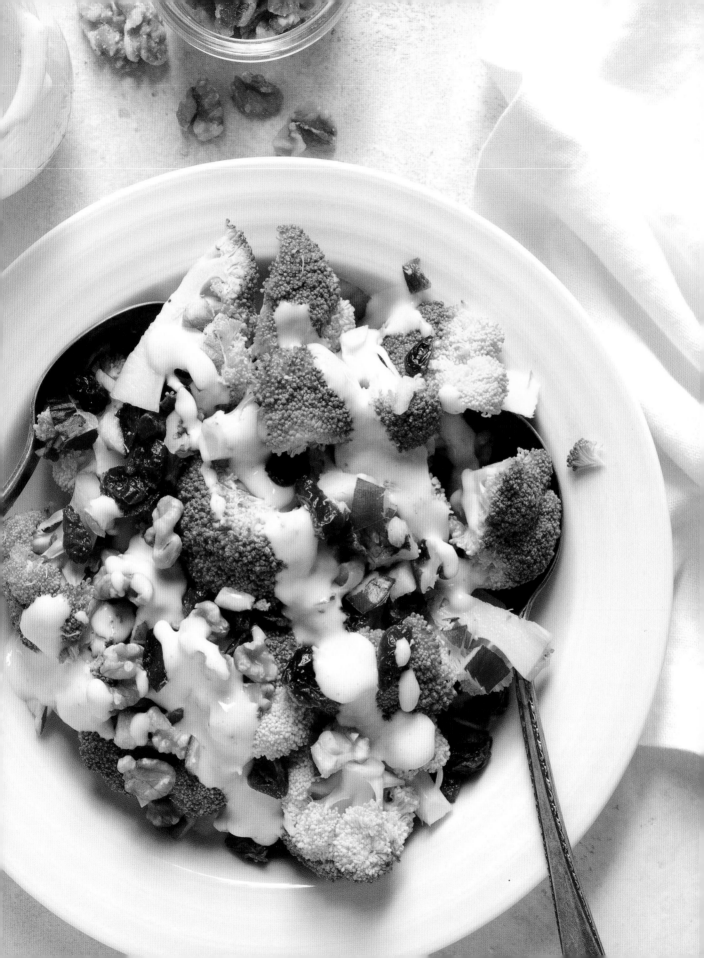

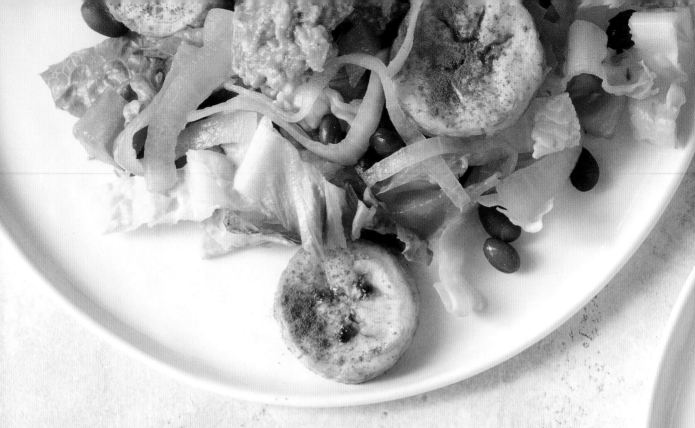

CARIBBEAN SALAD WITH GUACAMOLE

MAKES 6 CUPS

Baked sweet plantains sprinkled with cinnamon are a wonderful addition to green salads, especially when prepared with tomatoes, onions, black beans, and guacamole. I generally like this salad without dressing, but I do squeeze a bit of lemon juice on top.

4 cups chopped romaine lettuce

2 cups diced tomatoes

1 cup cooked or canned black beans

1 cup sliced onions

2 tablespoons vegetable broth

1½ cups *Plátanos Maduros* (page 267)

1 cup *Guacamole* (page 121)

Lemon juice and salt, to taste

1. Add lettuce, tomatoes, and black beans to salad bowl.

2. Sauté onions in vegetable broth over medium-high heat until brown.

3. Add onions and maduros to salad bowl. Gently toss all ingredients together.

4. Top with guacamole. If desired, season with lemon juice and salt.

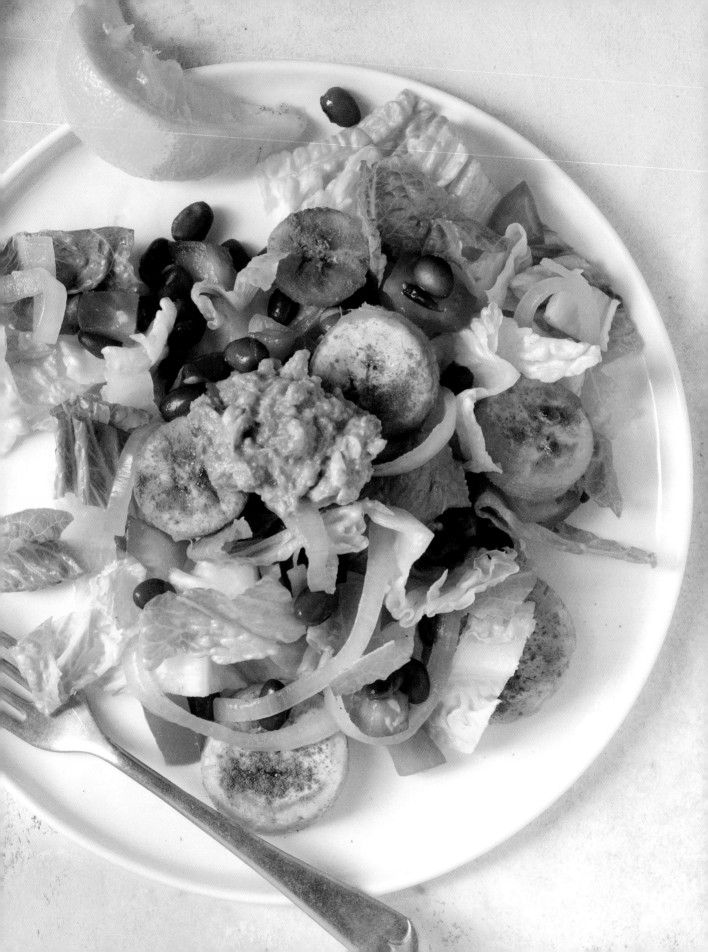

COLESLAWS

Coleslaws are wonderful side dishes that go well with wraps, sandwiches, baked potatoes, and burgers. I especially like to serve them with African Vegetables (page 192), Carrot Bake (page 202), Tomatillo Tortilla Bake (page 242), and Polenta Pie with Rice and Beans, Salsa, and Guacamole (page 232).

SIMPLE CABBAGE SLAW

MAKES 4 CUPS

3 cups grated cabbage

¼ cup grated carrots

½ cup grated red bell peppers

¼ cup diced dill pickles

2½ tablespoons rice vinegar

1 teaspoon agave

¼ cup *Golden Garden Mayonnaise* (page 184)

1 teaspoon dried dill

Salt and black pepper, to taste

1. Place cabbage, carrots, red bell peppers, and dill pickles in a bowl.

2. In a separate bowl, mix vinegar, agave, mayonnaise, and dill. Add to cabbage mixture and toss to mix.

3. Season with salt and black pepper.

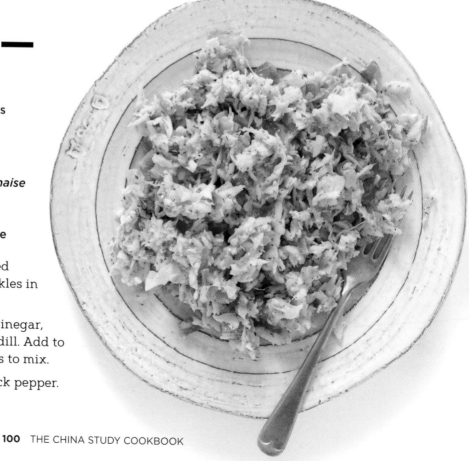

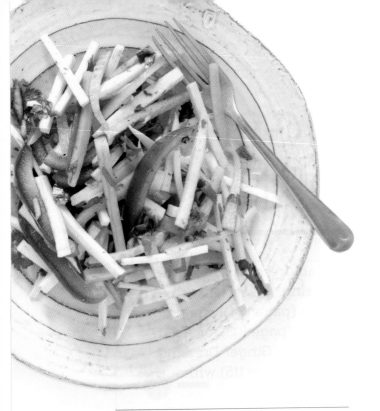

CARROT BEET SLAW

MAKES 4 SERVINGS

1 cup grated carrots

1½ cups grated beets

¼ cup grated onions

2 tablespoons *Lemon Tahini Dressing* (page 103)

¼ cup crushed peanuts

Salt and black pepper, to taste

Mix all ingredients together in a salad bowl.

JICAMA SLAW

MAKES 4–6 SERVINGS

1 cup julienned jicama root

1 cup julienned cucumber

¼ cup julienned green bell peppers

¼ cup diced red onion

¼ cup chopped fresh cilantro

⅛ teaspoon chili powder

2 tablespoons lime juice

Salt and cayenne pepper, to taste

Mix all ingredients together in a salad bowl.

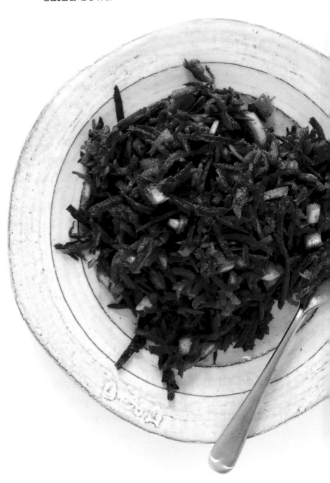

ENSALADA AZTECA

MAKES 8 CUPS

If I'm asked to bring a salad to an event or potluck, this is one of my "go-to" salads. Without fail, I always have several people asking for this recipe. The mango, lime, and ginger in the Mango Azteca Dressing (page 103) provide the perfect balance of sweet and sour.

2 (15-ounce) cans black beans, rinsed and drained

2 cups cooked quinoa or brown rice

½ cup finely chopped red onion

1 green bell pepper, seeded and diced

1 large tomato, diced

1 large avocado, pitted and diced

2 cups frozen corn, thawed

½ cup diced mango

1 jalapeño, minced

¾ cup chopped fresh cilantro

1 recipe *Mango Azteca Dressing* (page 103)

Salt, to taste

1. Combine beans, quinoa, onion, bell pepper, tomato, avocado, corn, mango, jalapeño, and cilantro in a large salad bowl.

2. Pour dressing over salad. Toss gently to mix. Season with salt.

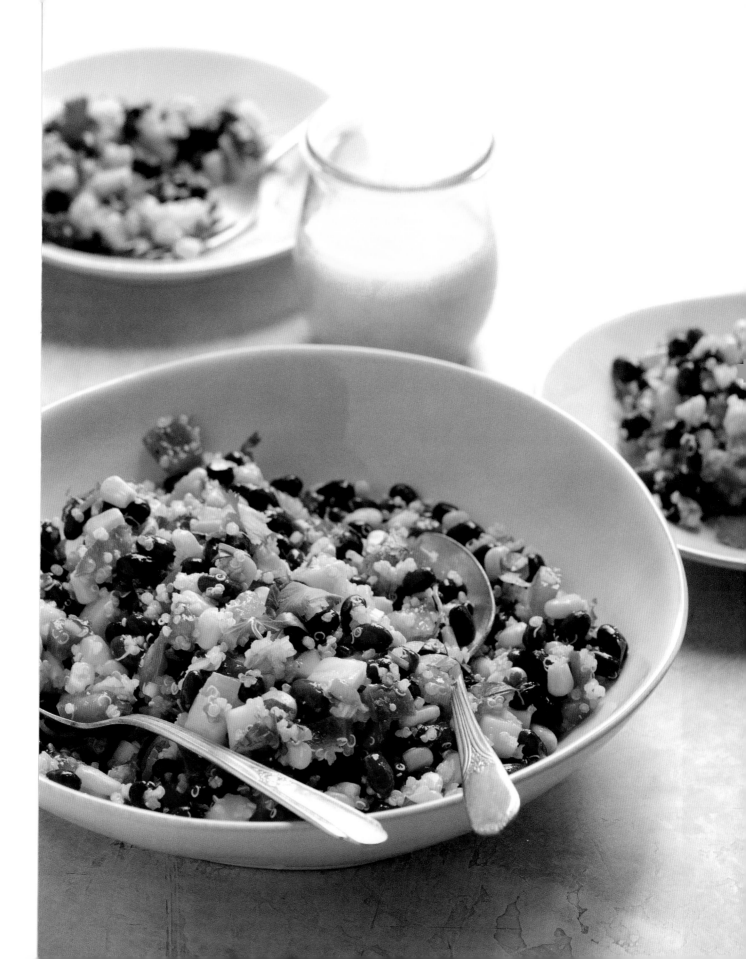

FRESH TOMATO AND AVOCADO PASTA SALAD

MAKES 4–6 SERVINGS

If you have Golden Garden Mayonnaise (page 184) or any other fat-free plant-based "mayo" on hand and want a quick pasta salad, this is a great one to make. It's easy and tasty, especially for those who like avocados. The chickpeas can be replaced with navy or cannellini beans.

—   —

3 cups cooked pasta shells

¼ cup diced red onion

2½ cups cherry tomatoes, quartered

2 avocados, pitted and diced

1½ cups frozen corn, thawed

1 (15-ounce) can chickpeas, rinsed and drained

2 teaspoons dried basil

¼ cup *Golden Garden Mayonnaise* (page 184)

½ teaspoon lemon juice

Salt, to taste

In a large bowl, combine all ingredients and toss well to mix.

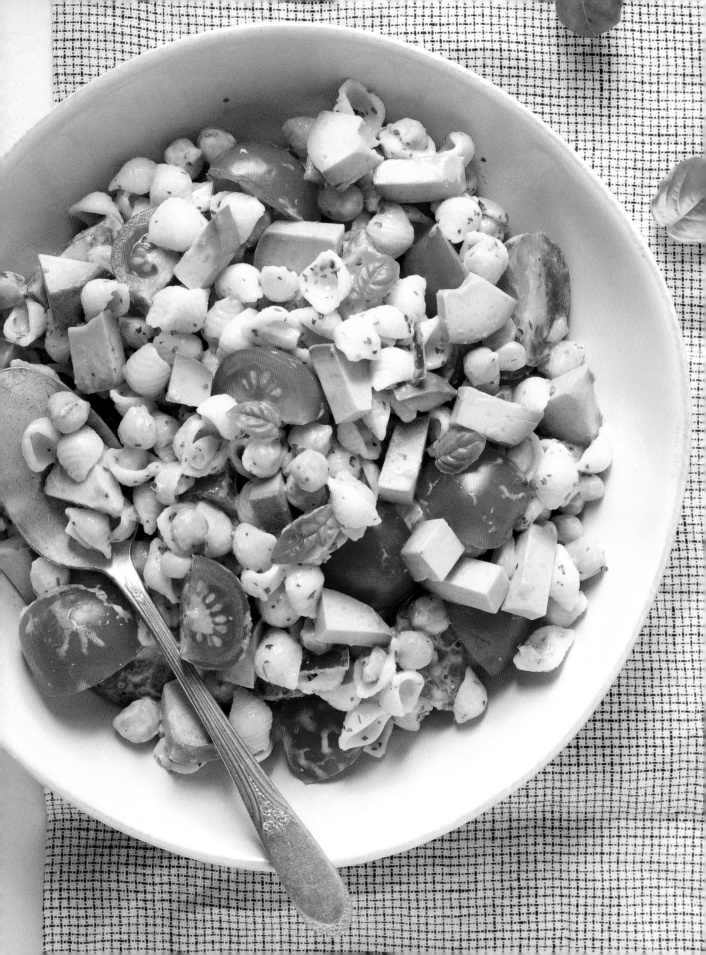

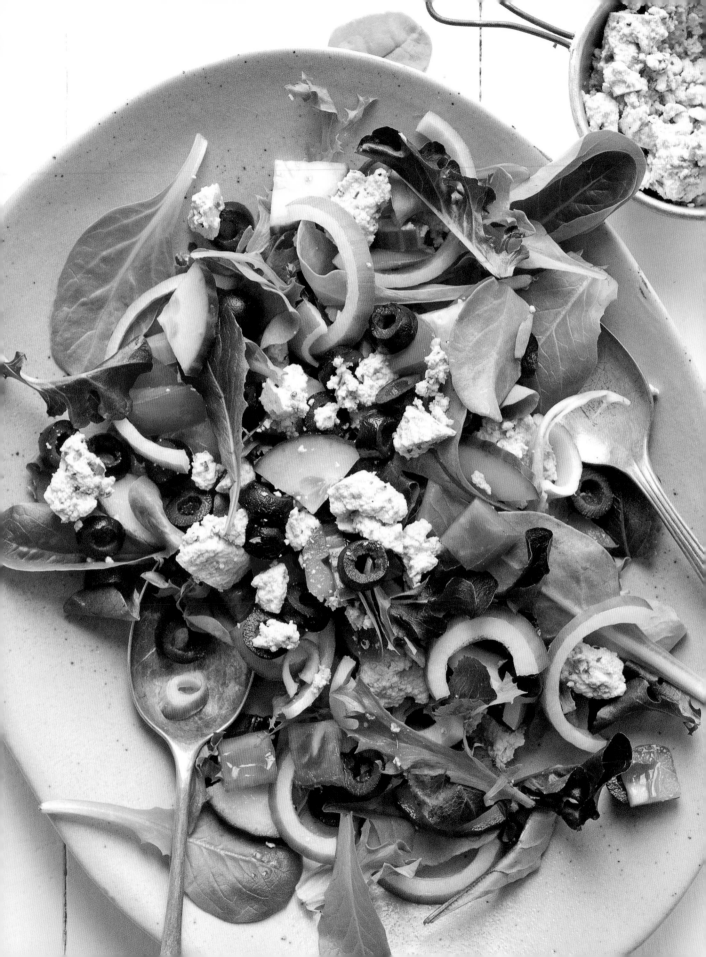

GREEK SALAD WITH TOFU "FETA"

MAKES 8½ CUPS

This Greek salad is great as a side with pizza and pasta. I also like serving it on its own with one of my favorite whole grain breads, especially Sensational Herb Bread (page 53). If I know I'm going to have leftovers, I don't add the tofu "feta" directly to the salad; instead, I add some to each serving. Then I refrigerate it separately so that the salad greens are not soggy the next day.

1 cup crumbled extra-firm tofu
½ cup red wine vinegar
1 teaspoon dried oregano
Salt and black pepper, to taste
6 cups salad greens
1 cup chopped cucumbers
1 cup diced tomatoes
½ cup diced red onions
½ cup chopped Kalamata olives

1. In a small bowl, mix together tofu, vinegar, oregano, salt, and black pepper. Place in the refrigerator to marinate for 1 hour.

2. Combine salad greens, cucumbers, tomatoes, onions, and olives in a large salad bowl and toss to combine.

3. Add marinated tofu to salad.

KALE SALAD WITH SWEET POTATOES

MAKES 4 SERVINGS

At times, I crave raw kale—especially this salad! The secret to making a good kale salad is to take the time to rub the kale back and forth between your hands until it is soft and slightly wilted. If you don't like massaging the kale, chop it into small pieces many times over.

Salad

1 large sweet potato, peeled and diced

8 large kale leaves

1 (15-ounce) can chickpeas, rinsed and drained

1 large tomato, diced

1 large green bell pepper, seeded and diced

½ onion, finely diced

½ cup dried cranberries or raisins

Salad Dressing

6 tablespoons seasoned rice vinegar

2 tablespoons water

1 teaspoon agave

2 heaping tablespoons nutritional yeast

¼ teaspoon salt

1. Preheat oven to 350°F. Line a baking sheet with parchment.

2. Spread out diced potatoes on lined baking sheet. Bake for 15–20 minutes. Set aside.

3. Tear the kale leaves from the stems into bite-size pieces. Rub the kale between your hands until soft and slightly wilted.

4. Put kale in a large salad bowl. Add chickpeas, tomato, bell pepper, onion, and dried cranberries and toss to combine.

5. In a separate bowl, whisk together all the salad dressing ingredients. Pour over the salad and serve.

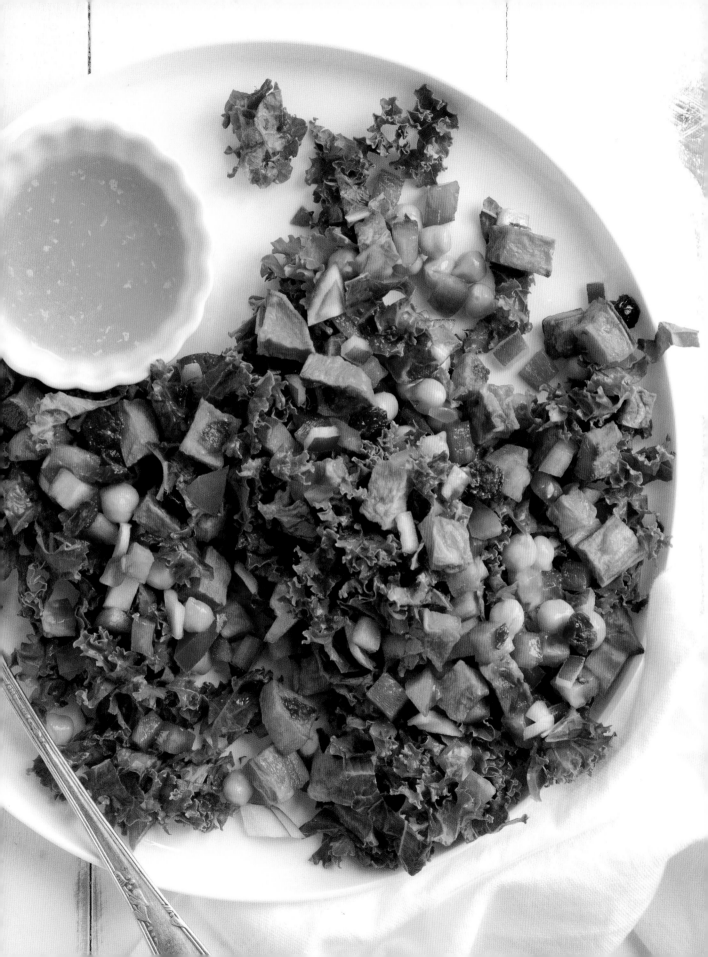

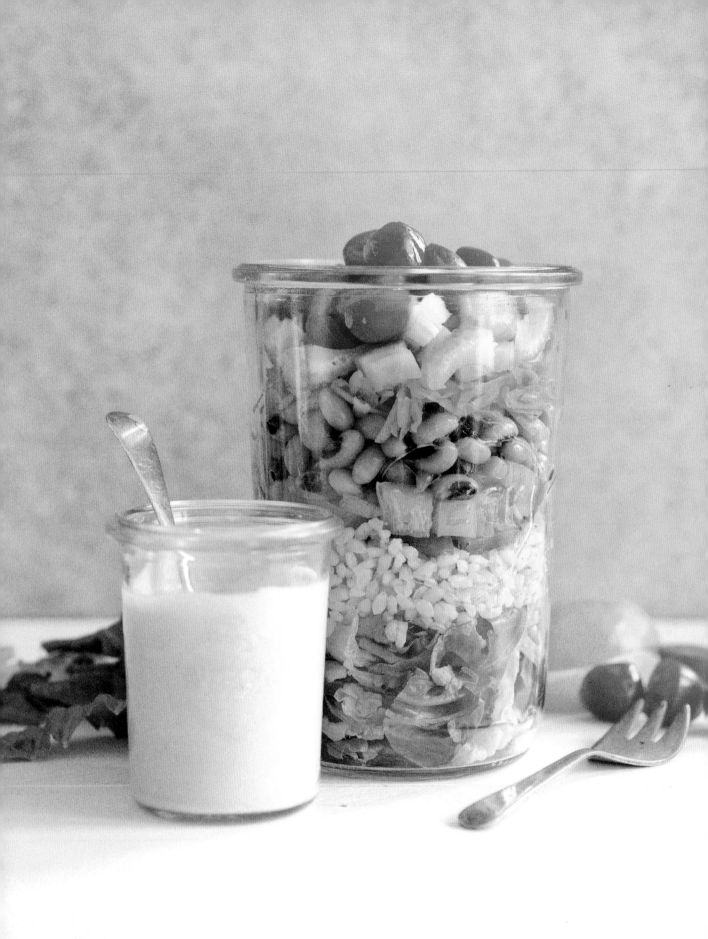

LAYERED BLACK-EYED PEA SALAD

MAKES 4-5 SERVINGS

Black-eyed peas are a Southern staple. They are traditionally served on New Year's Day to bring good luck. Compared to other legumes, I find black-eyed peas to have a nuttier taste. When I use them in salads, I like to add celery and tomatoes. In this recipe, they can be replaced with navy beans.

2 cups chopped romaine lettuce

2 cups cooked brown rice

1 cup chopped green and yellow bell peppers

2 cups cooked or canned black-eyed peas

½ cup grated carrots

½ cup diced celery

1 cup diced tomatoes

1 recipe *Lemon Tahini Dressing* (page 103)

In a large clear bowl, layer the salad ingredients in order: romaine lettuce, rice, bell peppers, black-eyed peas, carrots, celery, and tomatoes. Top with dressing.

LETTUCE WRAPS WITH PEANUT SAUCE

MAKES 4–5 WRAPS

I first had lettuce wraps in Chicago ten years ago. Since then, I've become a big fan of using lettuce or collard leaves to replace tortillas and sandwich bread. For the peanut sauce, I suggest using PB2 since it's considerably lower in fat than peanut butter. But if you don't have it on hand, replace the PB2 and water with 3 tablespoons of low-fat natural peanut butter.

4–5 large lettuce leaves (Bibb or romaine)

3 garlic cloves, minced

½ cup diced onions

½ cup grated carrots

¼ cup chopped celery

1 teaspoon dried thyme

2 tablespoons vegetable broth

1 cup diced canned water chestnuts

¼ cup reduced-sodium soy sauce

2 cups cooked grain (bulgur, brown rice, quinoa)

2 tablespoons nutritional yeast (optional)

Salt and black pepper, to taste

Peanut Sauce

¼ cup unsweetened nondairy milk (rice, soy, almond, etc.)

6 tablespoons PB2 whisked with 3 tablespoons water

2 tablespoons reduced-sodium soy sauce

1 tablespoon rice vinegar

½ teaspoon ground ginger

¼ teaspoon Sriracha (optional)

1. Wash lettuce leaves, pat dry, and set aside.

2. In a skillet, sauté garlic, onions, carrots, celery, and thyme in vegetable broth over medium heat for 3–5 minutes, until vegetables brown. Remove from heat.

3. Stir in water chestnuts, soy sauce, grain, and nutritional yeast (if using). Season with salt and black pepper.

4. Whisk together all the peanut sauce ingredients.

5. Place 2–3 tablespoons of the vegetable filling in the center of each lettuce leaf. Add 1 tablespoon peanut sauce. Roll into a wrap and enjoy.

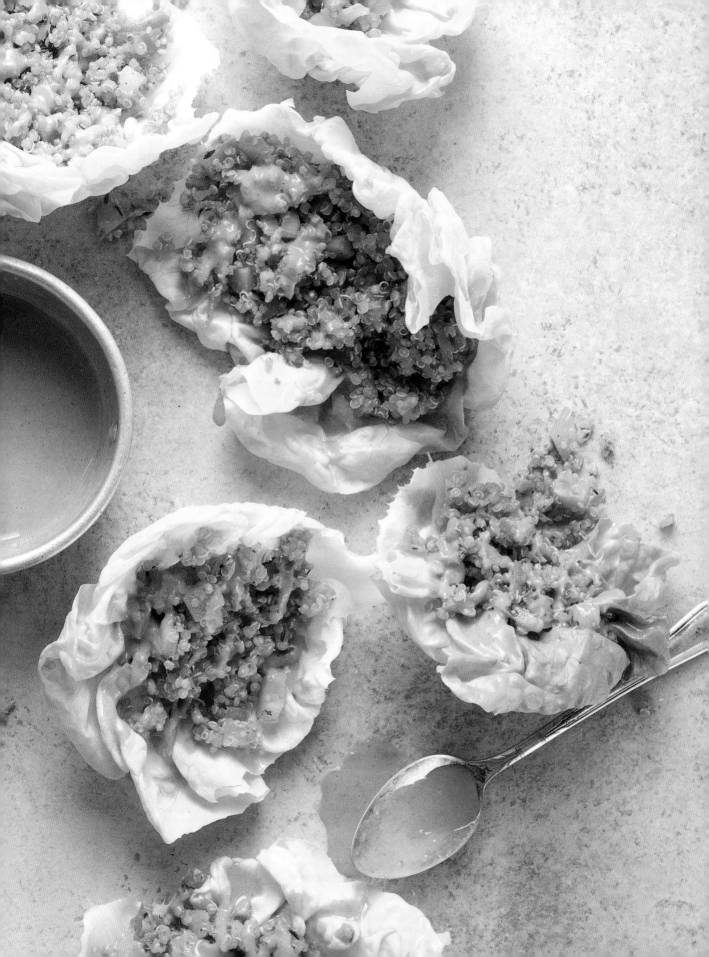

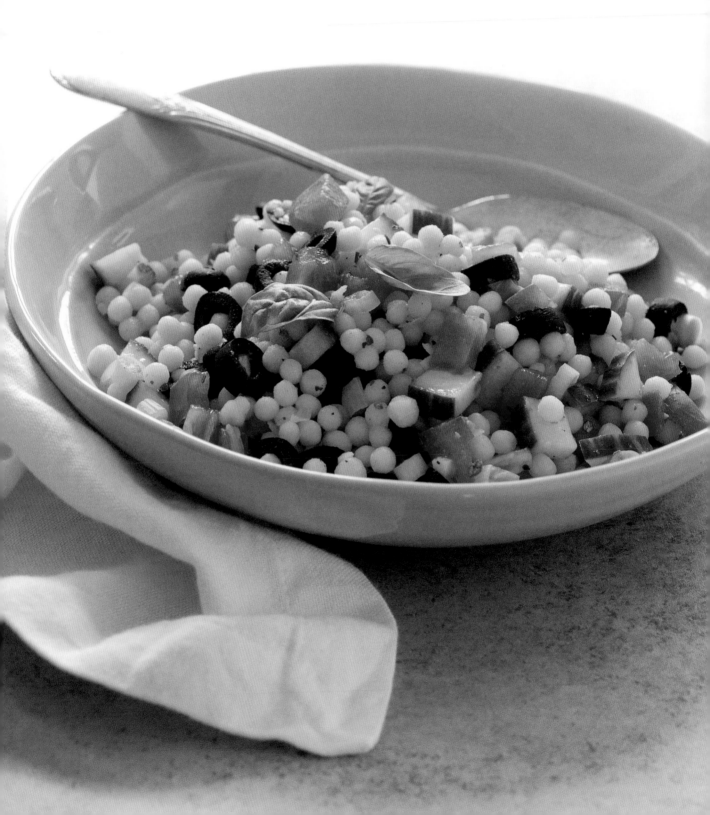

MEDITERRANEAN PEARL COUSCOUS

MAKES 4–6 SERVINGS

Pearl couscous (also known as Israeli couscous) is larger than regular couscous and has a chewy texture. It's a popular children's dish and can be prepared in lots of different ways.

2 tablespoons water

¼ cup chopped onions

2 garlic cloves, minced

2 cups vegetable broth

1 cup pearl couscous

1 cup chopped tomato

½ cup chopped cucumber

5 tablespoons chopped green onions

¼ cup chopped Kalamata olives

1 tablespoon chopped fresh basil

¾ teaspoon dried oregano

Sea salt and black pepper, to taste

1. In a saucepan, combine water, onions, and garlic. Cook over medium heat until onions brown.

2. Add vegetable broth and bring to a full boil over medium-high heat.

3. Stir in the couscous, then reduce heat to medium.

4. Simmer for 5–10 minutes, until couscous is tender.

5. Transfer cooked couscous to a serving bowl, then add the tomato, cucumber, green onions, olives, basil, and oregano. Toss well to combine. Season with salt and black pepper.

SALSA BAR AND GUACAMOLE

For this salsa bar, I've included a tomatillo sauce and a roasted tomato salsa. Both go well with baked chips, burritos, tostadas, and tacos (page 186). I have also included a basic ceviche recipe, which goes well with baked corn chips. For the guacamole recipe, I use either tomatillo sauce or roasted tomato salsa, then balance it with lemon and salt.

TOMATILLO SAUCE

MAKES 1½ CUPS

2 cups chopped tomatillos, husks
  removed
1 tablespoon lime juice
½ jalapeño, chopped
2 tablespoons chopped fresh cilantro
1 garlic clove, minced
2 tablespoons minced onion
Salt, to taste

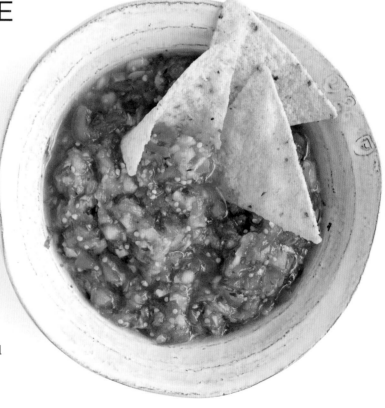

1. In small saucepan, combine tomatillos, lime juice, and jalapeño. Cook over medium heat until soft, 5–6 minutes.

2. Transfer tomatillo mixture to a food processor and add cilantro, garlic, and onion. Process until smooth.

3. Season with salt.

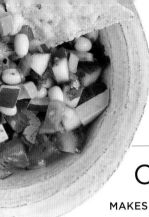
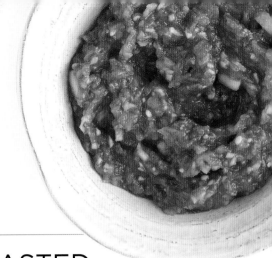

CEVICHE

MAKES 3 CUPS

1 medium red onion, diced
1 medium cucumber, diced
2 medium tomatoes, diced
¼ cup chopped fresh cilantro
1 (15-ounce) can white beans, rinsed and drained
1 avocado, pitted and diced
Juice of 2 limes
Salt, to taste
Baked corn chips, crumbled

1. Combine onion, cucumber, tomatoes, and cilantro in a medium-size bowl.

2. Mix in beans, avocado, and lime juice. Season with salt.

3. Top with crumbled corn chips.

GUACAMOLE

MAKES 2 CUPS

2 avocados
¼ cup *Roasted Tomato Salsa* or ¼ cup *Tomatillo Sauce*
Lemon juice and salt, to taste

1. Scoop avocado flesh into a medium-size bowl and mash with a fork.

2. Stir in salsa or tomatillo sauce. Season with lemon juice and salt. Mix well.

ROASTED TOMATO SALSA

MAKES 2 CUPS

1½ cups chopped tomatoes
2 garlic cloves
¼ cup chopped onions
1½ tablespoons lemon juice
2 tablespoons chopped jalapeño
2 tablespoons chopped fresh cilantro
¼ teaspoon ground cumin
¼ teaspoon chili powder
Salt, to taste

1. Preheat oven to 400°F. Place tomatoes and garlic cloves on a parchment-lined baking sheet and cook for 45–50 minutes.

2. Place tomatoes, garlic, and remaining ingredients in a food processor and pulse 5–6 times, until blended but still chunky.

3. Adjust seasonings if necessary.

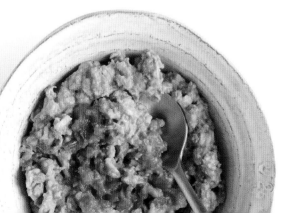

SAMOSAS BAKED TO PERFECTION

MAKES 16 SAMOSAS

These stuffed pastries are a favorite in Indian cuisine. Most samosas are deep-fried, but in this recipe, I bake the samosas, then top them with a Creamy Dijon Sauce (page 274).

1½ cups warm water

1 tablespoon raw cane sugar

2½ teaspoons instant (rapid-rise) yeast

3½ cups whole wheat pastry flour

½ teaspoon sea salt

1 cup diced onions

2 garlic cloves, minced

1 teaspoon ground coriander

1 teaspoon ground cumin

½ teaspoon ground turmeric

1 teaspoon fennel seeds

4 tablespoons vegetable broth, divided

3 cups diced cooked potatoes

1 cup cooked green peas

1 teaspoon sea salt

1 cup *Creamy Dijon Sauce* (page 274), for serving

1. For the dough, mix water, sugar, and yeast in a large bowl. Let sit for 2–3 minutes.

2. Add flour and salt. Knead with your hands for 8–10 minutes, until smooth and elastic. Divide into 16 balls. Cover and let rise for 45 minutes.

3. While the dough is rising, prepare filling. In a medium-size skillet, sauté onions, garlic, coriander, cumin, turmeric, and fennel seeds in 1 tablespoon of vegetable broth over medium-high heat for 2–3 minutes, until onions brown.

4. Add remaining 3 tablespoons of vegetable broth, potatoes, peas, and salt. Cover and cook for 3–5 minutes. Set aside. Preheat oven to 400°F.

5. Roll out each dough ball to a circle 3 inches in diameter. Place 1½ tablespoons filling in the center. Fold dough over and pinch edges together. There should be no openings along the edge. Place on a parchment-lined baking sheet.

6. Bake for 15 minutes, until lightly brown.

7. Serve with Dijon sauce.

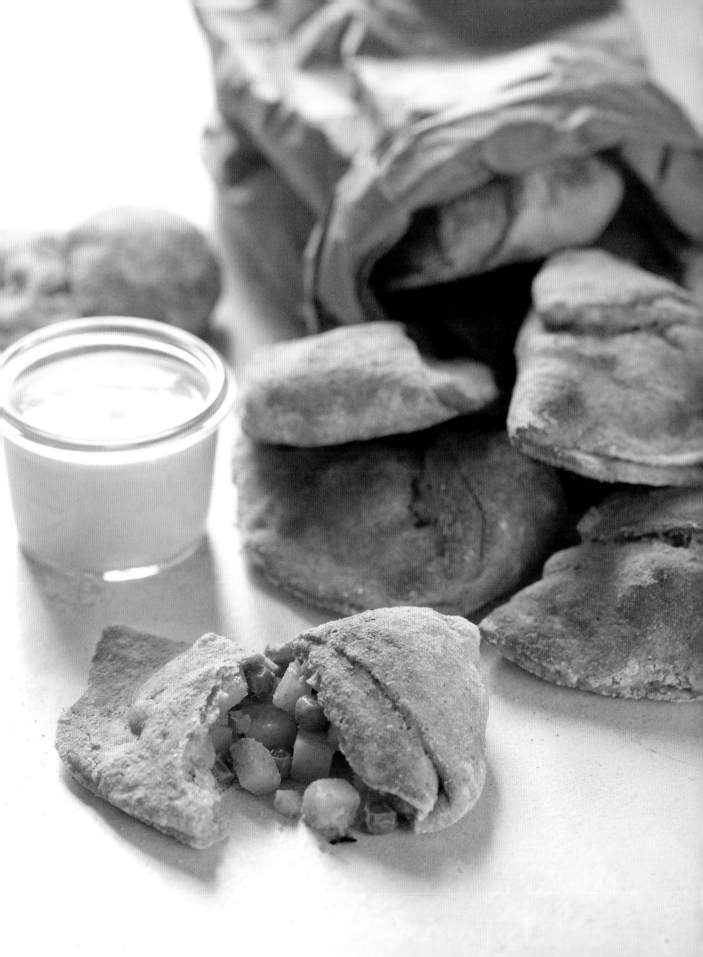

SAVORY ROASTED VEGETABLES WITH CUCUMBER DILL DIP

MAKES 3 CUPS VEGETABLES AND 2 CUPS DIP

This simple appetizer goes well with both fresh vegetables and roasted vegetables. When roasting vegetables, I like to add an Italian herb seasoning, but you can also use garlic powder, onion powder, or lemon pepper seasoning.

1 large russet potato, cut into bite-size pieces

1 large sweet potato, cut into bite-size pieces

1 bunch broccoli, cut into bite-size pieces

1 cup green beans, cut in half

1 tablespoon Italian seasoning

Sea salt and black pepper, to taste

Cucumber Dill Dip

1 cup silken tofu or drained *Yogurt* (page 84)

1 tablespoon lemon juice

3 garlic cloves

½ teaspoon salt

2 teaspoons fresh dill

1 cup cucumbers, grated

2 tablespoons green onions, chopped

Black pepper, to taste

1. Preheat oven to 400° F. Line a baking sheet with parchment.

2. Spread vegetables on lined baking sheet. Sprinkle with Italian seasoning, sea salt, and black pepper.

3. Bake for 20–25 minutes, until crunchy.

4. Meanwhile, make cucumber dill dip. In a food processor, blend tofu, lemon juice, garlic, salt, and dill. Pour into a small bowl.

5. Fold in cucumbers and green onions , then season with black pepper.

6. Serve vegetables with dip.

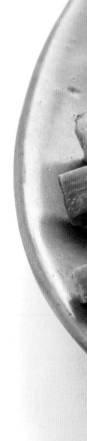

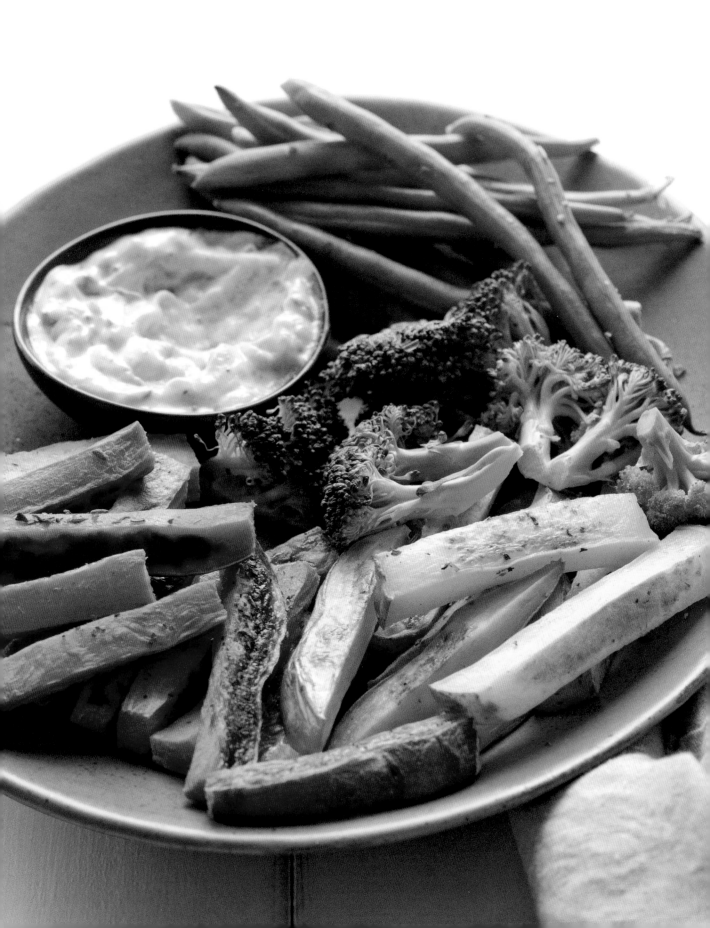

SOUTHWESTERN SALAD

MAKES 10 CUPS

This is one of my son's favorite salads. The black beans and corn are cooked with oregano, garlic, and salt, then tossed with fresh vegetables and crushed tortilla chips. We often skip the salad dressing and enjoy it as is.

1 cup cooked or canned black beans

1 cup corn

1 teaspoon dried oregano

½ teaspoon garlic powder

½ teaspoon salt

6 cups salad greens

1 small red onion, diced

1 green bell pepper, seeded and diced

1 avocado, pitted and diced

2 medium tomatoes, diced

1–2 cups crushed baked tortilla chips

1 recipe salad dressing of your choice (optional)

1. In a small skillet, heat black beans, corn, oregano, garlic powder, and salt over medium heat.

2. Meanwhile, mix salad greens, onion, bell pepper, avocado, and tomatoes in a large salad bowl.

3. Add bean mixture to the salad, then top with crushed tortilla chips. If desired, add the dressing.

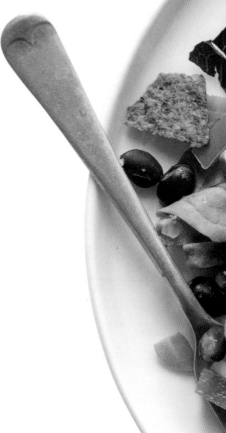

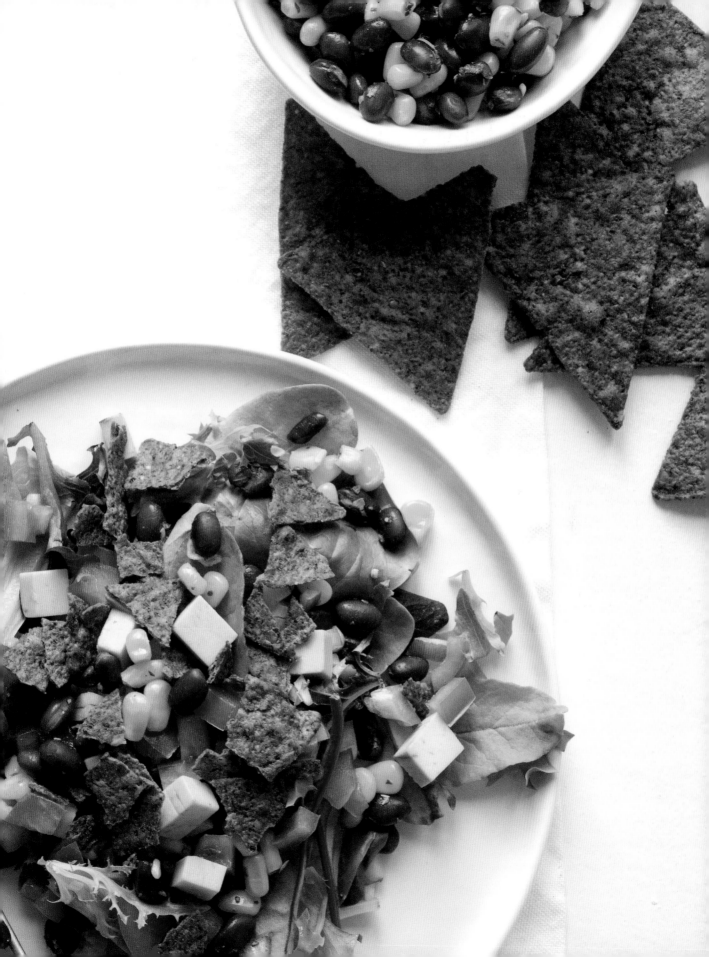

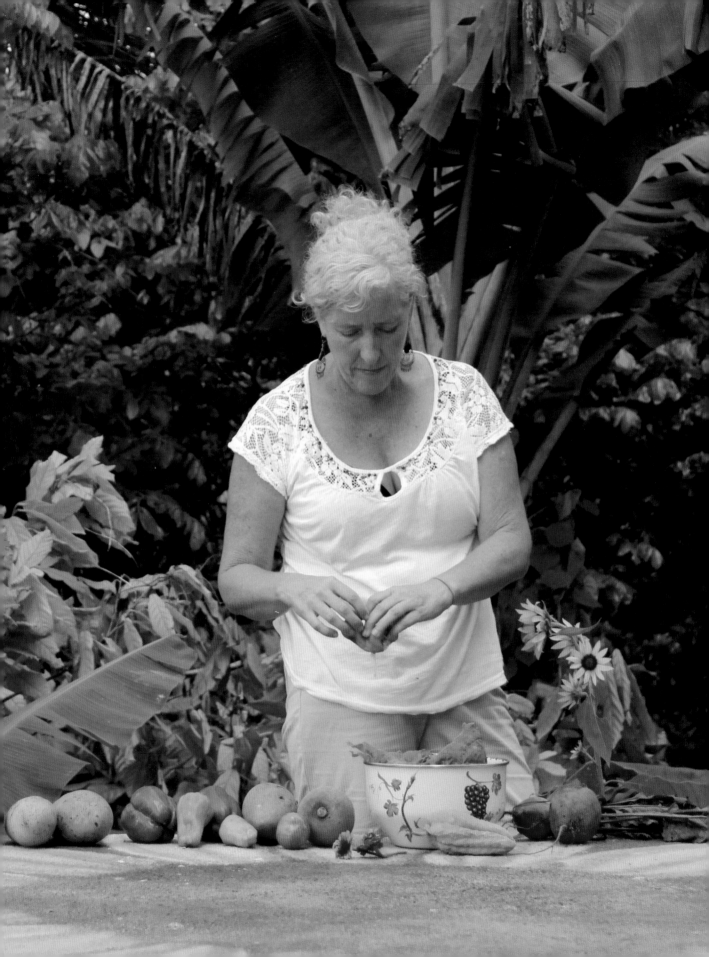

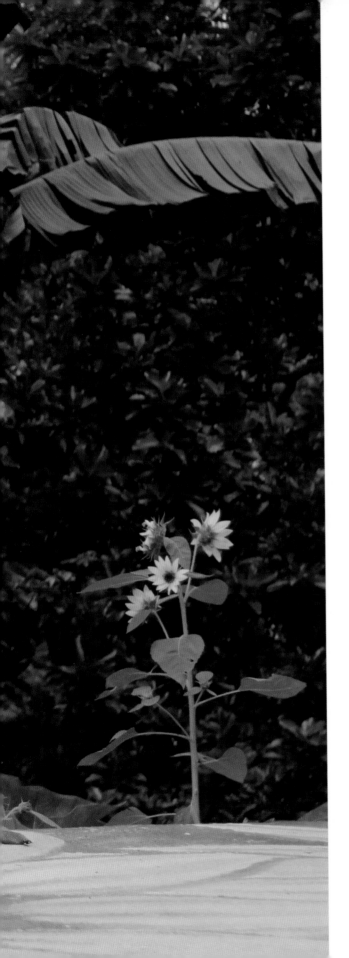

SOUPS

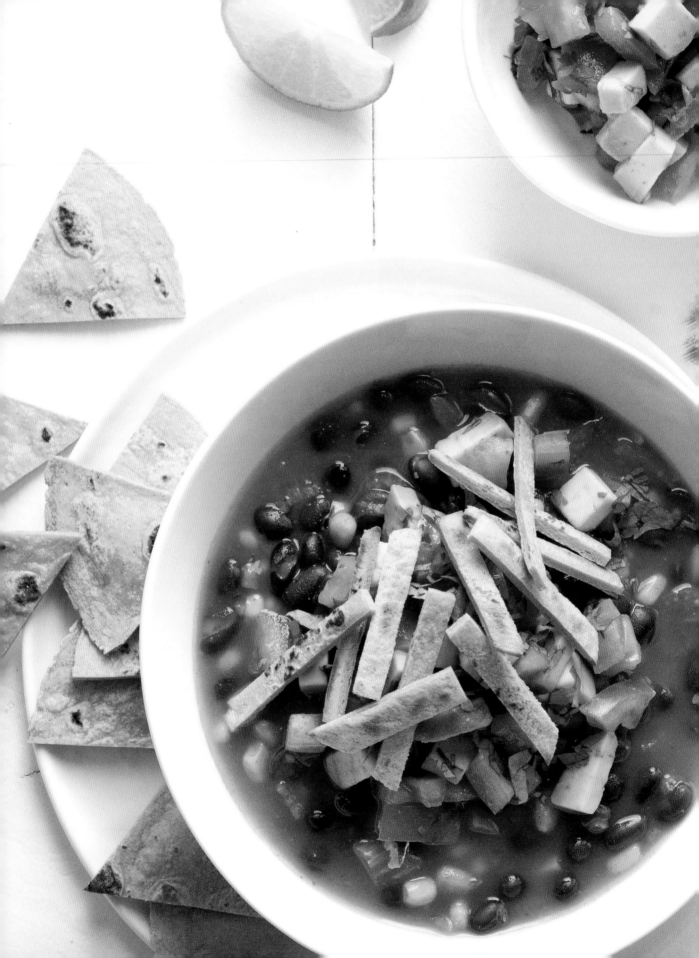

AZTEC SOUP

MAKES 3-4 SERVINGS

I first had a version of this soup in the beautiful city of Mérida, Mexico, and I loved it—especially the intensity of flavors and the toppings. It's typically made with chicken stock, then topped with fried tortilla strips. However, I'm using vegetable broth and baked corn tortillas. In addition to the tortilla strips, make sure to top it with avocados and tomatoes.

6 corn tortillas

¾ cup diced onion

4 garlic cloves, minced

½ cup diced celery

3 cups plus 2 tablespoons vegetable broth, divided

1 cup corn

2 (15-ounce) cans black beans, rinsed and drained

2 teaspoons ground cumin

1 teaspoon smoked paprika

¼ teaspoon cayenne pepper

2 tablespoons lime juice

Sea salt and black pepper, to taste

1 avocado, pitted and diced

1 medium tomato, diced

¼ cup chopped fresh cilantro

1. Preheat oven to 300°F.

2. Place corn tortillas on a baking sheet and sprinkle with salt. Bake for 10–12 minutes, until crispy.

3. Meanwhile, in a large saucepan, sauté onion, garlic, and celery in 2 tablespoons of vegetable broth over medium-high heat until onion browns. Add corn, beans, cumin, paprika, and cayenne pepper. Cook for 3–4 minutes.

4. Add remaining vegetable broth and lime juice. Bring to a boil, then reduce heat and simmer for 3–5 minutes. Season with salt and black pepper.

5. In a bowl, combine avocado, tomato, and cilantro.

6. Pour hot soup into bowls and garnish with avocado mix and crumbled baked tortillas.

CABBAGE CARAWAY SOUP

MAKES 4 SERVINGS

This is what I refer to as "anytime soup" because I nearly always have this combination of vegetables on hand. But if you don't, you can substitute other vegetables, like sweet potatoes or butternut squash in place of the potatoes and cauliflower in place of the cabbage. Just remember, keep the same combination of herbs and it will come out good every time.

1 cup chopped onions
1 cup diced carrots
⅓ cup diced celery
1 garlic clove, minced
4 cups vegetable broth, divided
3 cups thinly sliced cabbage
2 cups diced potatoes
2 teaspoons dried dill
¼ teaspoon ground caraway seeds
½ teaspoon paprika
½ teaspoon salt
¼ teaspoon black pepper

1. In a large saucepan, sauté onions, carrots, celery, and garlic in 2 tablespoons of vegetable broth over medium-high heat until onions brown.

2. Add cabbage and cook for an additional 1–2 minutes.

3. Add remaining vegetable broth, potatoes, dill, caraway, paprika, salt, and black pepper. Cover and bring to a low boil. Cook for 25–30 minutes, until potatoes are tender.

4. Remove from heat and serve immediately.

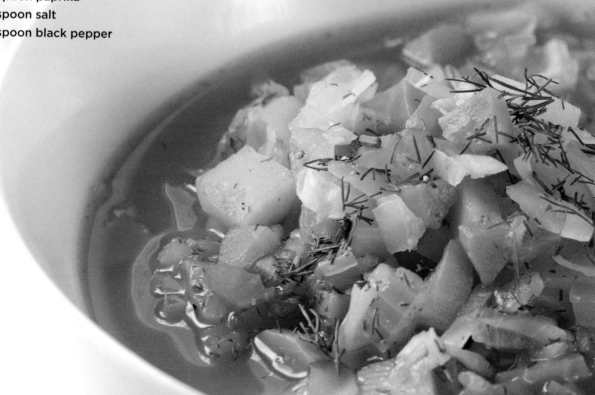

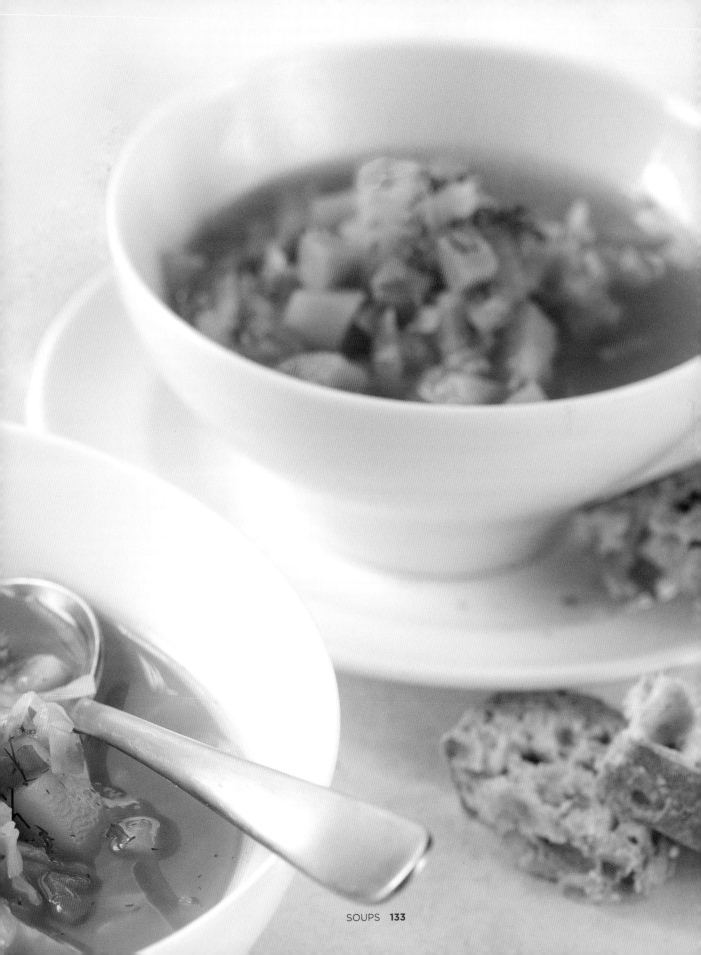

COCONUT CORN CHOWDER

MAKES 3-4 SERVINGS

This simple, flavorful chowder gets its richness from coconut milk. Since coconut milk has a high fat content, I suggest using lite coconut milk; you can also try almond milk.

1 medium leek, chopped

3 garlic cloves, minced

1 jalapeño, minced

4–5 small potatoes, thinly sliced

2 cups vegetable broth, divided

1 (15-ounce) can garbanzo beans, rinsed and drained

1 cup corn

1 (14-ounce) can lite coconut milk

Salt and red pepper flakes, to taste

1. In a soup pot, sauté leek, garlic, jalapeño, and potatoes in ½ cup of vegetable broth over medium-high heat until vegetables are tender, about 5 minutes.

2. Add garbanzo beans, corn, coconut milk, and remaining 1½ cups of vegetable broth. Bring to a boil. Lower temperature, cover, and simmer for 8–10 minutes, until potatoes become soft.

3. Season with salt and red pepper flakes.

4. Serve hot.

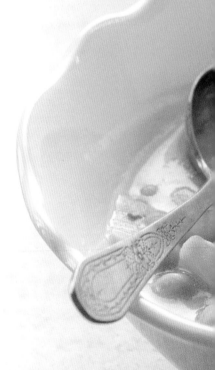

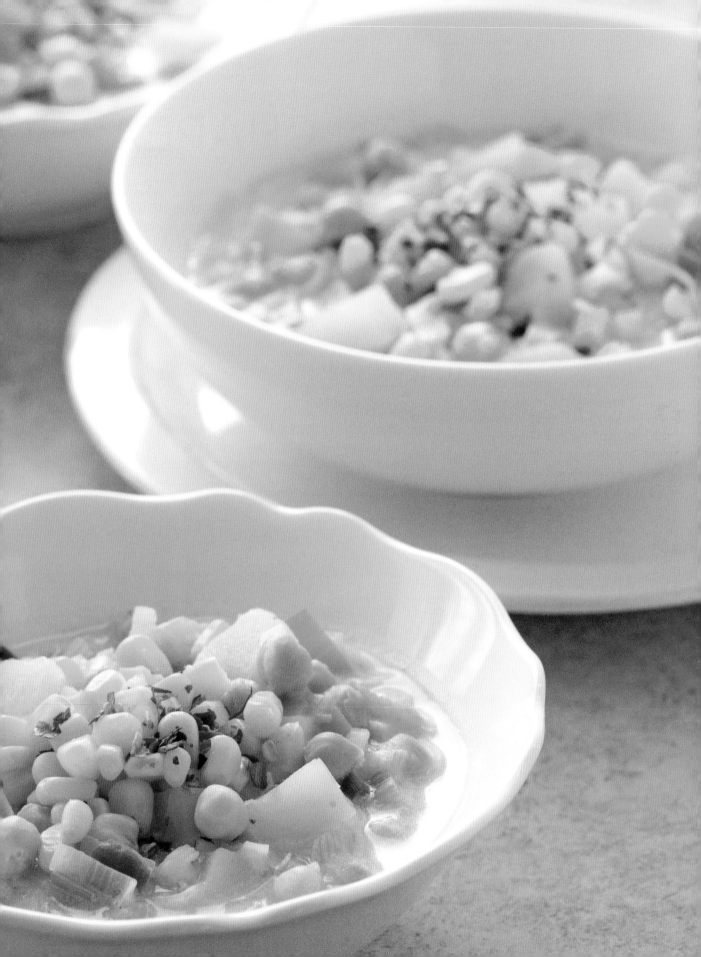

DOMINICAN CHAPEA

MAKES 6 SERVINGS

When I'm in the Dominican Republic, this is one of my favorite stews to make. Chapea tastes different in each house—some like it with chayote squash instead of butternut squash (pumpkin); others add broccoli or green plantains and skip the carrots. But what's common in every stew is the rice and beans, together with onions, garlic, bell peppers, and cilantro.

¼ cup minced onion

5 garlic cloves, minced

½ green bell pepper, minced

2 cups vegetable broth, divided

3 cups water

1 cup uncooked rice

¼ cup grated carrots

1½ cups chopped cauliflower

2 cups cooked or canned pinto beans

1½ cups diced butternut squash

¼ cup chopped fresh cilantro

1 tablespoon lemon juice

Salt and black pepper, to taste

1. In a large saucepan, sauté onion, garlic, and bell pepper in 2 tablespoons of vegetable broth until browned.

2. Add water and remaining vegetable broth and bring to a boil. Add rice, carrots, cauliflower, beans, and squash. Reduce heat to low, cover, and cook for 20 minutes.

3. Add cilantro and lemon juice. Cover and cook for an additional 5 minutes. Season with salt and black pepper.

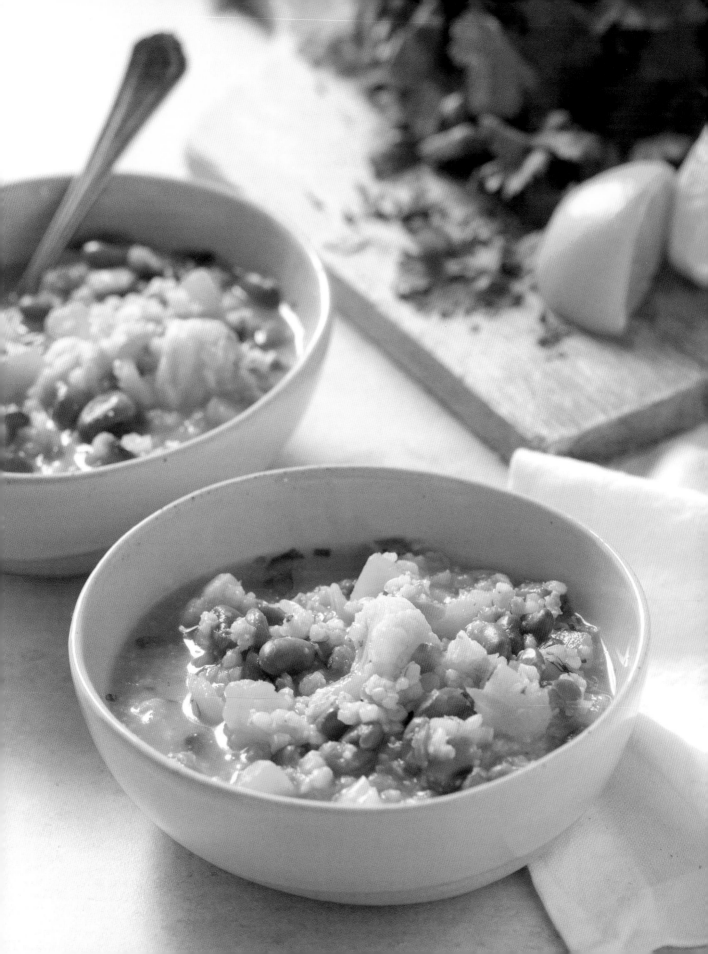

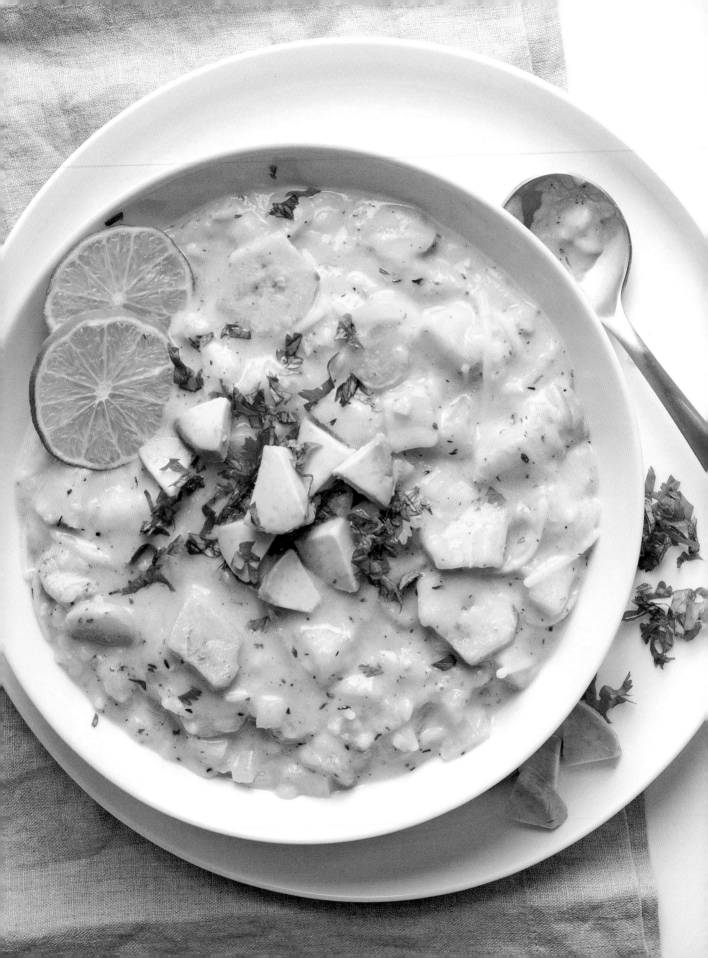

GREEN BANANA CASSAVA SOUP

MAKES 4 SERVINGS

In the Dominican Republic, green bananas are served nearly every day with meat and/or avocados. They also make a wonderful addition to soups. In this recipe, I have skipped the meat, added cassava (another traditional Dominican root crop), and topped it with diced avocado and sliced limes. It's one of my favorites!

½ cup diced onions

4 garlic cloves, minced

1 cup chopped carrots

⅓ cup chopped celery

2 tablespoons vegetable broth

6 cups water

1 cup canned lite coconut milk

2 bay leaves

2 teaspoons dried thyme

3 green bananas or plantains, peeled and chopped

1½ cups cassava, peeled and diced

1 teaspoon salt

½ teaspoon black pepper

½ cup whole wheat angel hair pasta, broken into 1-inch pieces

Garnish

1 tablespoon chopped fresh cilantro

Diced avocado

Sliced limes

1. In a large saucepan, sauté onions, garlic, carrots, and celery in vegetable broth over medium-high heat until onions brown.

2. Add water, coconut milk, bay leaves, and thyme. Bring to a boil.

3. Add bananas, cassava, salt, and black pepper. Simmer for 15 minutes.

4. Add angel hair pasta and cook for an additional 10 minutes, until vegetables are cooked.

5. Garnish with cilantro, diced avocado, and sliced limes.

HEARTY SALSA STEW

MAKES 4–6 SERVINGS

When I was younger my mother's friend used to pile vegetables in a casserole dish, add chicken and salsa, and then bake it. I loved it. I've tried to replicate the simplicity of this dish without the chicken and without baking it.

1 cup chopped onion

1 cup chopped red bell peppers

4 garlic cloves, minced

2 tablespoons vegetable broth

4 cups water

2 cups diced butternut squash

1 cup diced potatoes

1 (15-ounce) jar medium-hot salsa

1 (15-ounce) can crushed tomatoes

1 tablespoon dried oregano

2 zucchinis, chopped

1 (15-ounce) can pinto beans, rinsed and drained

1½ cups corn

1 tablespoon soy sauce, plus more to taste

Salt and black pepper, to taste

1. In a large soup pot, sauté onion, bell peppers, and garlic in vegetable broth over medium-high heat for 3–4 minutes, until onion browns.

2. Add water, butternut squash, potatoes, salsa, tomatoes, and oregano. Cover and simmer until squash is tender, about 15 minutes.

3. Add zucchini, pinto beans, and corn. Continue cooking for another 10 minutes. Add soy sauce, salt, and black pepper. Serve warm.

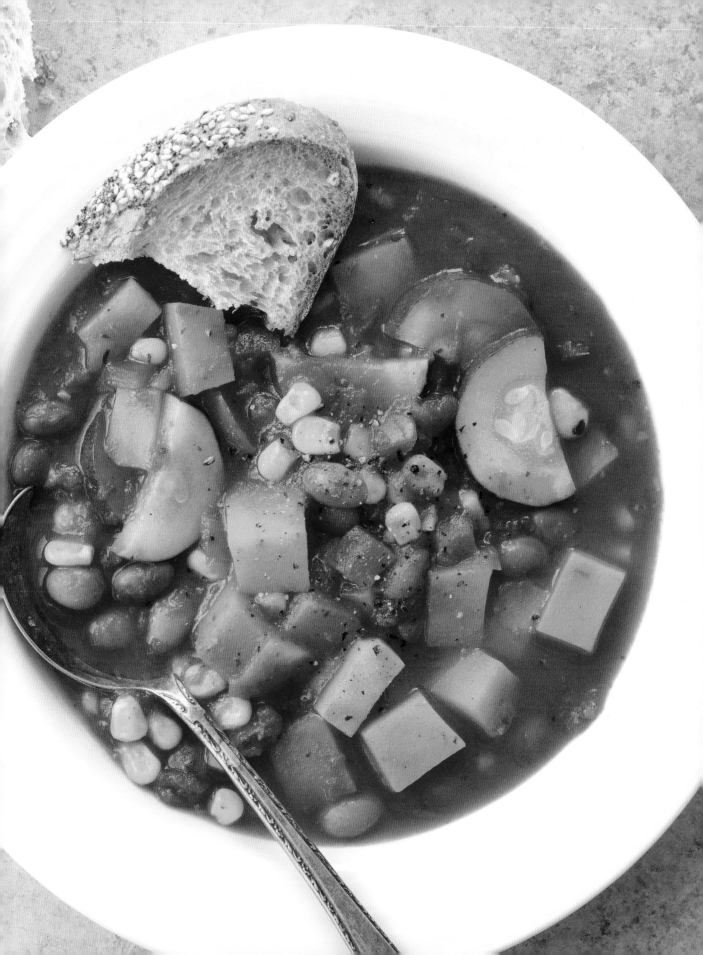

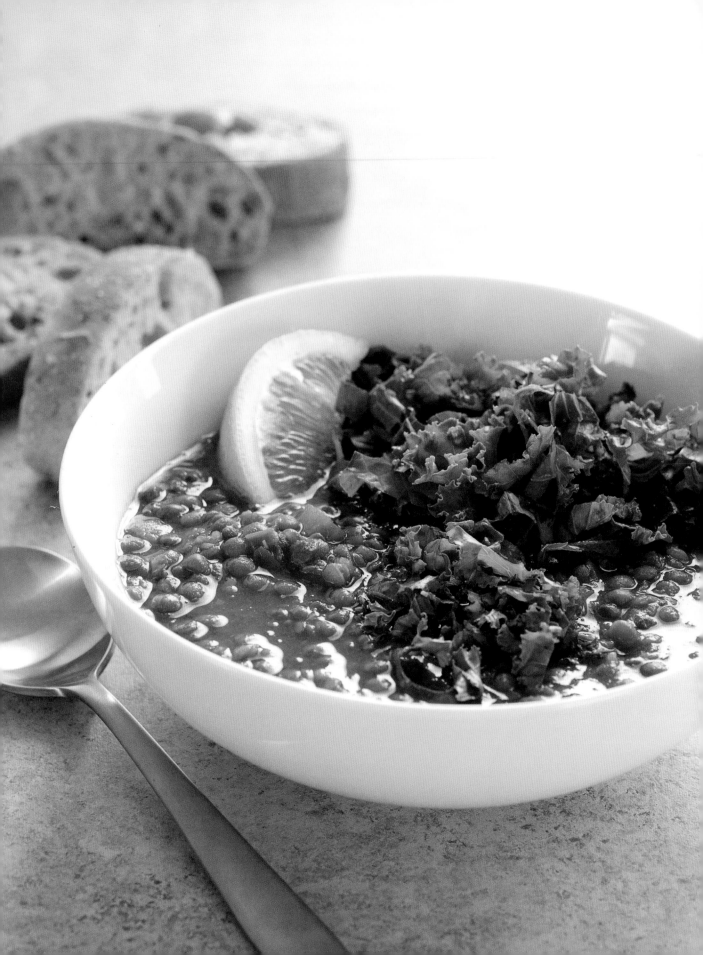

LENTIL SOUP: DELICIOUS, SIMPLE, AND EASY

MAKES 4-6 SERVINGS

When cooking lentils, take care not to overcook them—they are a lot better when they keep their shape. And if you're substituting red or yellow lentils for the brown lentils, you'll need to reduce the cooking time. If you want to make this soup heartier, add potatoes or one of your favorite greens (kale, spinach, or collards).

½ cup chopped onions

¼ cup chopped celery

4 garlic cloves, minced

4 cups vegetable broth, divided

2 teaspoons ground cumin

1 teaspoon curry powder

½ teaspoon dried thyme

2 cups diced tomatoes

2 cups brown lentils, picked over and rinsed

4 cups water

1 teaspoon salt, plus more to taste

¼ teaspoon red pepper flakes

1 teaspoon lemon juice, plus more to taste

Black pepper, to taste

1. In a large soup pot, sauté onions, celery, and garlic in 2 tablespoons of vegetable broth over medium-high heat for 3–4 minutes, until onions brown.

2. Add cumin, curry powder, and thyme. Cook until fragrant, stirring constantly, about 30 seconds.

3. Add diced tomatoes, lentils, water, remaining vegetable broth, salt, and red pepper flakes. Bring to a boil, then partially cover the pot and reduce heat to maintain a gentle simmer. Cook for 30 minutes, until lentils are tender but still hold their shape.

4. Remove the pot from heat and stir in the lemon juice. Taste and season with more salt, black pepper, and/or lemon juice. Serve immediately.

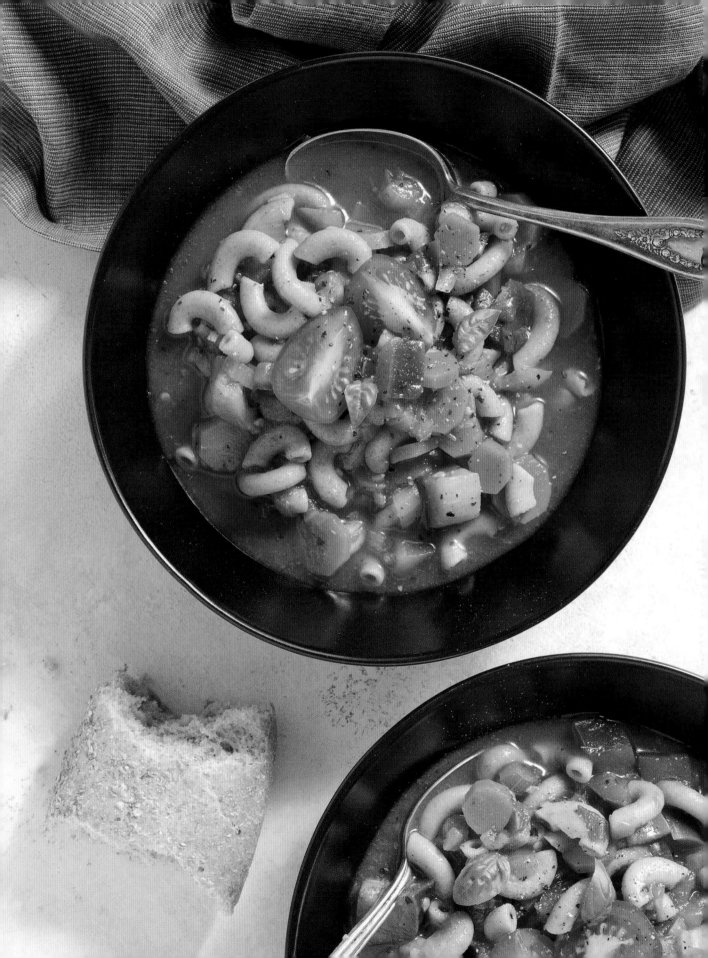

MACARONI EGGPLANT SOUP

MAKES 3-4 SERVINGS

Eggplants are one of my favorite vegetables. They are incredibly versatile and go especially well with tomatoes, potatoes, carrots, cauliflower, peas, and spinach. They add a nice addition to this Italian soup, complementing the basil, oregano, and macaroni. So if I'm having a pasta craving and I want something light, I make this soup. It hits the spot every time.

½ cup chopped onions

2 garlic cloves, minced

1 tablespoon vegetable broth

2 cups diced eggplant

¾ cup diced carrots

¼ cup diced celery

3 cups diced tomatoes

3 cups water

1 teaspoon raw cane sugar

1 teaspoon salt

½ teaspoon black pepper

½ teaspoon dried basil

½ teaspoon dried oregano

½ teaspoon ground allspice

½ cup uncooked macaroni

1. In a large saucepan, sauté onions and garlic in vegetable broth over medium-high heat until onions brown.

2. Add eggplant, carrots, celery, and tomatoes. Cover and cook for 5 minutes.

3. Add water, sugar, salt, black pepper, basil, oregano, allspice, and macaroni. Bring to a low simmer and cook until macaroni is soft.

4. Serve immediately.

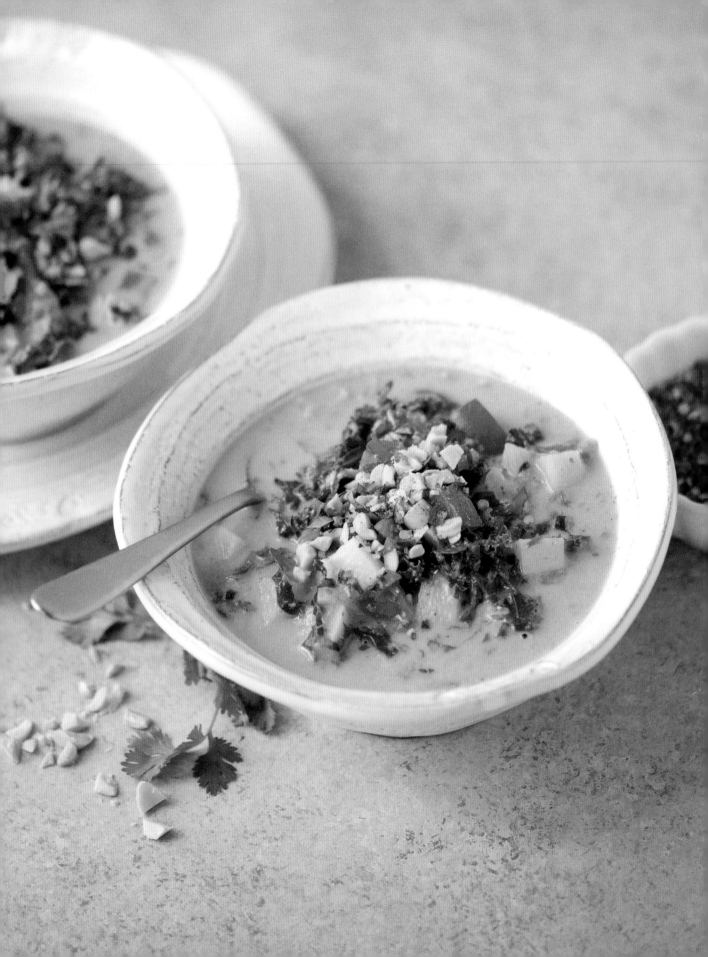

PEANUT KALE SOUP

MAKES 3-4 SERVINGS

Whenever I make this soup, I double it—and even then we eat almost all of it. It's one of those soups where everyone goes back for seconds, thirds, and yes, sometimes fourths. If I don't have kale on hand, I use collard greens or spinach.

1 cup diced onions

4 garlic cloves, minced

1 cup chopped red bell peppers

2 tablespoons vegetable broth

5 cups water

1½ cups diced potatoes

1 cup diced tomatoes

½ cup natural peanut butter

3 cups chopped kale

¼ teaspoon red pepper flakes

Salt, to taste

2 tablespoons chopped fresh
   cilantro, for garnish

¼ cup crushed peanuts,
   for garnish

1. In a large saucepan, sauté onions, garlic, and bell peppers in vegetable broth over medium-high heat, until onions brown.

2. Add water, potatoes, tomatoes, peanut butter, kale, and red pepper flakes. Bring to a boil, then lower heat and simmer for 8–10 minutes.

3. Season with salt and garnish with cilantro and crushed peanuts.

QUICK THREE-BEAN SOUP

MAKES 4–6 SERVINGS

My sons were raised on this soup. I often made it in the slow cooker before going to work by simply throwing everything into the pot, setting it on high, and then cooking it for 5–6 hours. When my older son went off to college, he asked for a slow cooker so he could make this soup.

1 medium onion, diced

4 garlic cloves, minced

3 cups vegetable broth, divided

1 (15-ounce) can black beans, rinsed and drained

1 (15-ounce) can kidney beans, rinsed and drained

1 (15-ounce) can chickpeas, rinsed and drained

1 (14-ounce) can crushed tomatoes with jalapeños

2 cups mixed vegetables (corn, chopped green beans, and/or chopped carrots)

1 teaspoon paprika

1 teaspoon black pepper

1 heaping teaspoon dried parsley

1 teaspoon dried oregano

Chopped fresh parsley, for garnish

1. In a large soup pot, sauté onion and garlic in 2 tablespoons of vegetable broth over medium-high heat until onion is slightly transparent.

2. Add remaining ingredients. Cover and cook over medium-low heat for 20–25 minutes. Garnish with fresh parsley.

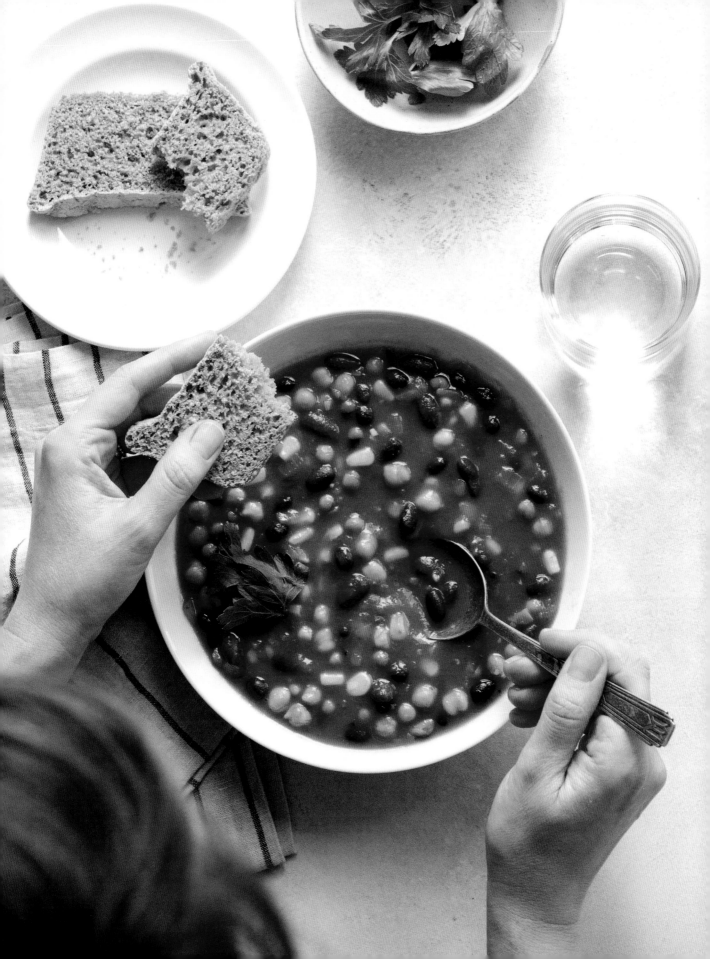

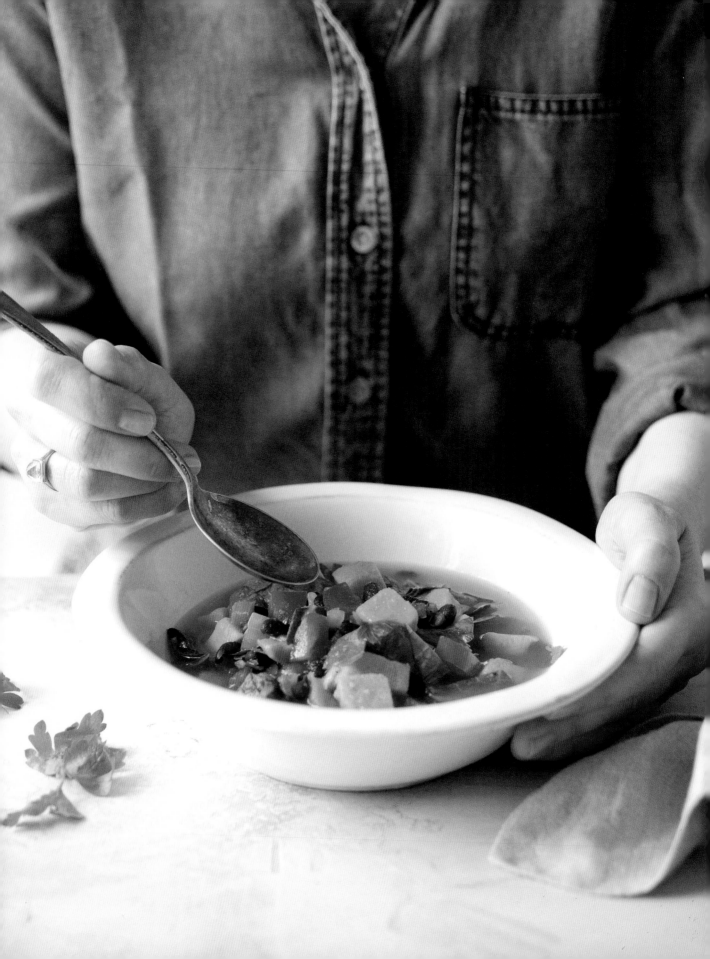

SCRUMPTIOUS SWEET POTATO, BLACK BEAN, AND COLLARD SOUP

MAKES 4 SERVINGS

You can't go wrong with this combination: sweet potatoes, black beans, and greens. What's nice about this recipe is that it takes only 15 minutes to make. It goes especially well with Sensational Herb Bread (page 53) and Avocado Hummus Wraps (page 177).

¾ cup chopped onions

¾ cup chopped red bell peppers

2 tablespoons vegetable broth

2 teaspoons ground cumin

2 teaspoons curry powder

1 (15-ounce) can black beans, rinsed and drained

4 cups water

1 large sweet potato, peeled and diced

4 cups chopped collard greens

¾ teaspoon salt

½ teaspoon black pepper

1. In a soup pot, sauté onions and bell peppers in vegetable broth over medium-high heat until brown. Stir in cumin and curry powder and cook for 1–2 minutes.

2. Add beans, water, potatoes, collard greens, salt, and black pepper. Cover and simmer for 8–10 minutes.

SEASONED BARLEY MUSHROOM SOUP

MAKES 3-4 SERVINGS

I love cooking with barley. Its rich, nutty flavor and chewy, pasta-like consistency go well in soups, especially mushroom soups. When choosing barley, try to find the hulled variety rather than the pearl version since the hulled variety is less processed. Pearl barley is golden brown, whereas hulled barley is light brown.

1 cup chopped onions
4 garlic cloves, minced
1 medium carrot, chopped
4 cups vegetable broth, divided
2 cups sliced white button or
   baby portobello mushrooms
1 teaspoon dried thyme
1 bay leaf
2 cups water
1 cup barley
½ teaspoon salt
Black pepper, to taste
1 teaspoon red wine vinegar

1. In a soup pot, sauté onions, garlic, and carrot in 2 tablespoons of vegetable broth over medium-high heat for 3–5 minutes, until onions brown.

2. Add mushrooms, thyme, and bay leaf. Cook for 1 minute.

3. Add remaining vegetable broth, water, and barley. Bring to a simmer, cover, and cook for about 45 minutes, until the barley is tender.

4. Season with salt and black pepper. Stir in vinegar.

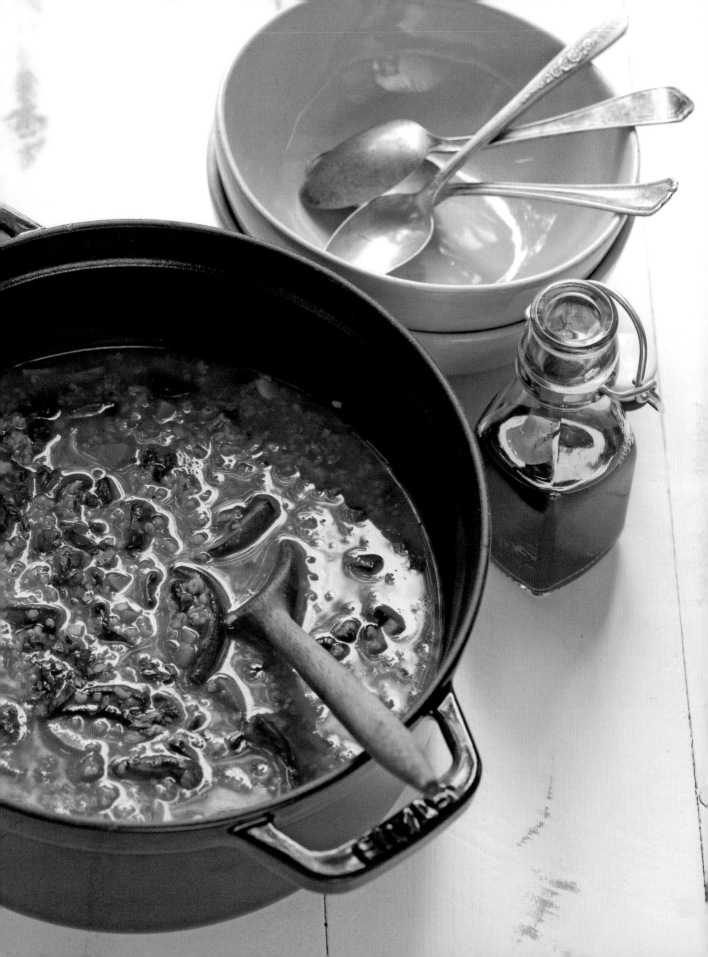

SPICY PUMPKIN SOUP

MAKES 4 SERVINGS

This wonderfully versatile squash can be prepared in many different ways, including Pumpkin Gnocchi with Italian Vegetable Sauce (page 234), Pumpkin Pie Muffins with Pecans (page 42), Pumpkin Pancakes (page 78), Quick and Easy Pumpkin Pie (page 309), and even savory soups. Creamy and flavorful, this soup can be made in 20 minutes.

½ cup chopped onions

1 garlic clove, minced

2 teaspoons grated fresh ginger

2 tablespoons vegetable broth

½ teaspoon curry powder

½ teaspoon ground cumin

½ teaspoon ground coriander

⅛ teaspoon red pepper flakes

1½ cups canned lite coconut milk

2 cups water

1 cup diced potatoes

½ cup cooked or canned
  white beans

1 (15-ounce) can pumpkin puree

Salt, to taste

Toasted pumpkin seeds,
  for garnish

1. In a large saucepan, sauté onions, garlic, and ginger in vegetable broth over medium-high heat for 3–5 minutes, until onions brown.

2. Add curry powder, cumin, coriander, and red pepper flakes. Cook for 1 minute.

3. Add coconut milk, water, potatoes, beans, and pumpkin puree. Bring to a simmer. Cover and cook for 15–20 minutes, until potatoes are tender.

4. Season with salt and garnish with toasted pumpkin seeds.

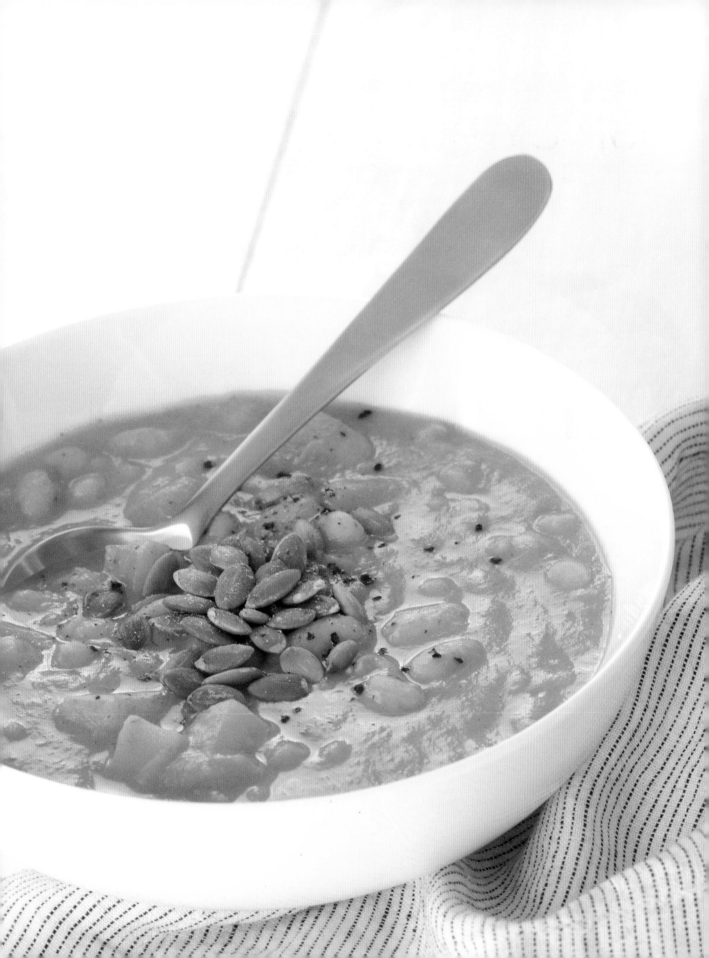

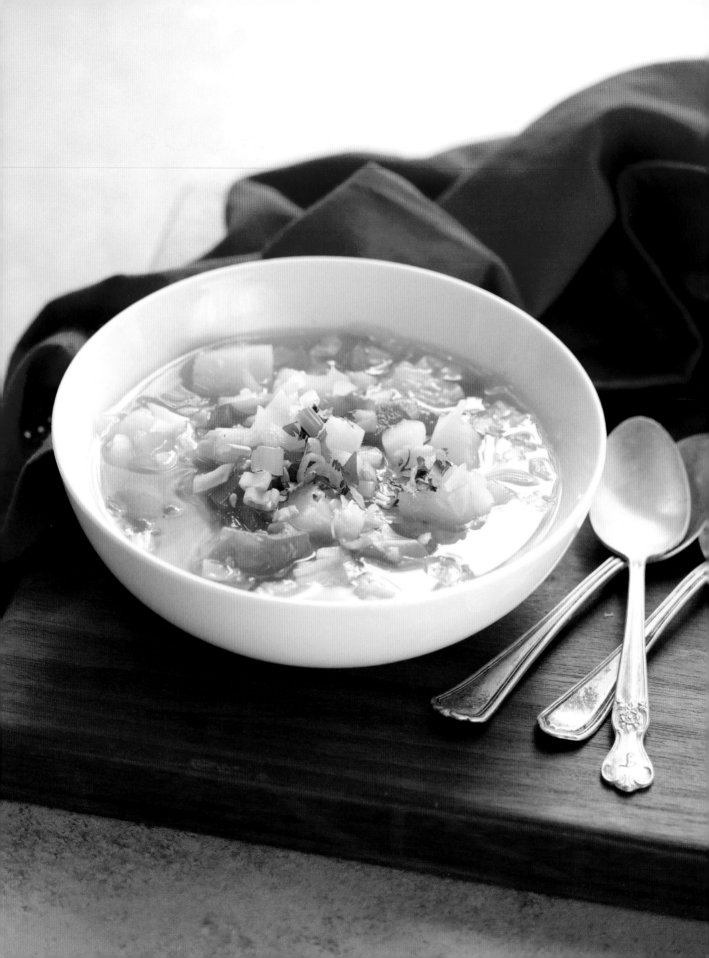

SWEET AND SOUR FUSION

MAKES 3-4 SERVINGS

A mixture of flavors, this is one of my dad's favorite soups. A version of this soup is served in Vietnamese restaurants and is known as canh chua. It's generally cooked with fish sauce and tamarind paste (which is difficult to find in my local grocery store). I've tweaked the soup a bit, and it's still delicious.

1½ cups chopped cabbage

¼ cup finely chopped onions

2 garlic cloves, minced

2 tablespoons vegetable broth

4 cups water

3 tablespoons lime juice

3-4 tablespoons raw cane sugar

1½ teaspoons salt

½ teaspoon hot sauce (such as Sriracha)

1 cup chopped pineapple

1 cup chopped tomato

2 tablespoons minced green onion, for garnish

2 tablespoons chopped fresh cilantro, for garnish

1. In a large saucepan, sauté cabbage, onions, and garlic in vegetable broth over medium-high heat, until onions brown.

2. Add water, lime juice, sugar, salt, and hot sauce. Taste and adjust seasonings if needed. Bring to a boil and simmer for 2–3 minutes.

3. Add pineapple and tomato. Cook for an additional 1–2 minutes.

4. Garnish with green onions and cilantro. Serve immediately.

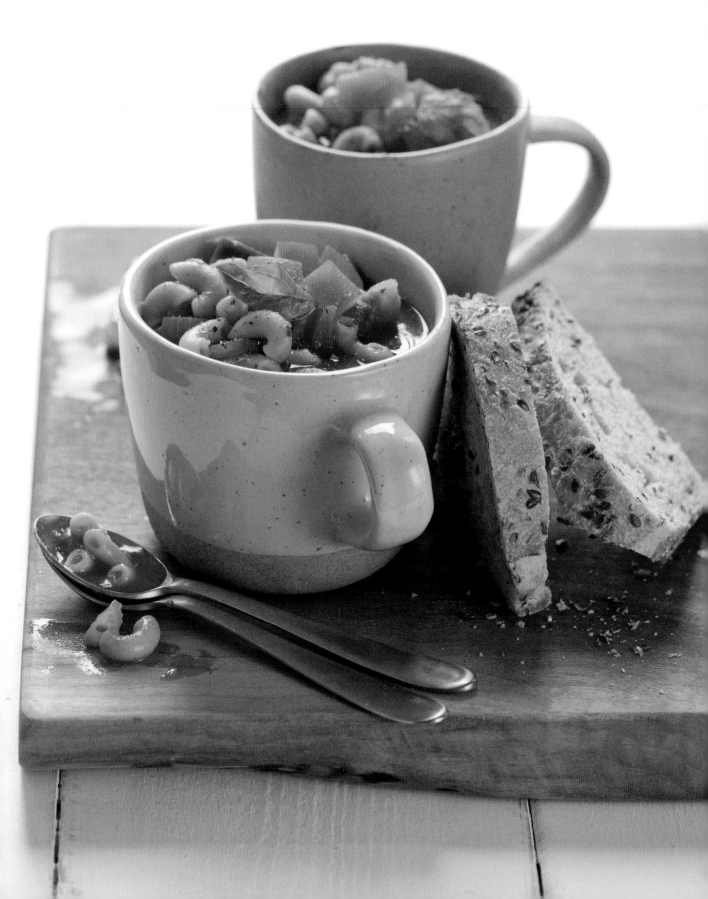

TOMATO PASTA SOUP

MAKES 4 SERVINGS

I love pasta, especially in this flavorful tomato soup. In this recipe, I recommend farfalline, a small version of farfalle, or bow-tie pasta. However, you can use just about any small pasta shape; if using spaghetti, break it into small pieces. I like to use a whole wheat or rice pasta.

1 cup chopped onions

4 garlic cloves, minced

2 teaspoons minced jalapeños

1½ cups vegetable broth, divided

1 (28-ounce) can diced tomatoes

1½ cups water

½ cup uncooked farfalline or other small pasta

1 teaspoon dried basil

1 teaspoon dried oregano

1 teaspoon salt

½ cup corn

1 cup diced zucchini

Black pepper, to taste

1. In a large soup pot, sauté onions, garlic, and jalapeños in 2 tablespoons of vegetable broth over medium-high heat until onions begin to brown.

2. Add tomatoes with their juice, remaining vegetable broth, water, and pasta. Bring to a simmer, then reduce heat and add basil, oregano, salt, corn, and zucchini. Cover and cook for 8–10 minutes, until pasta is cooked.

3. Season with black pepper.

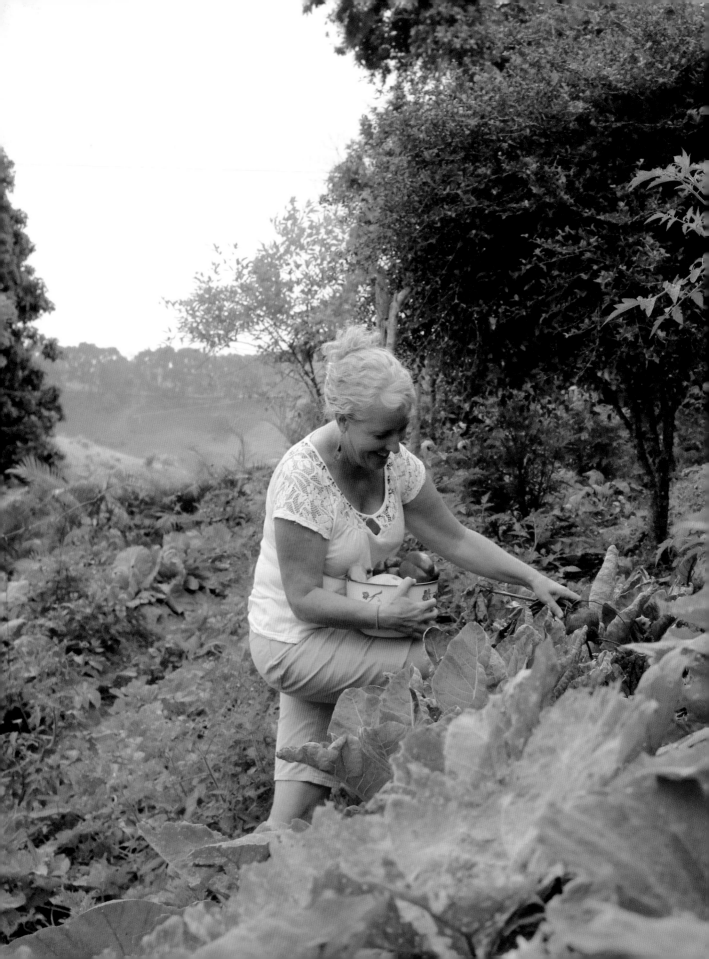

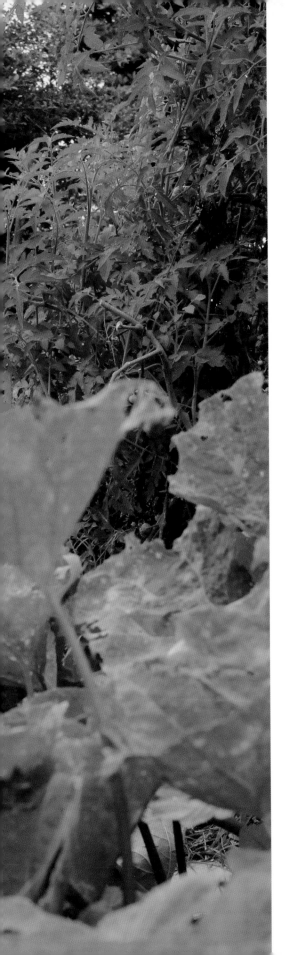

SANDWICHES AND **WRAPS**

BAKED FALAFEL IN PITA

MAKES 4 PITAS

Chickpeas are a staple in my household. I always have a couple of cans on hand to use in some of my favorite quick recipes: Coconut Corn Chowder (page 134), Hummus (pages 176–177), Ocean Chickpea Sandwiches (page 178), Quick Three-Bean Soup (page 148), Masala's Chickpeas (page 218), and this falafel, which is especially good with shredded lettuce and Cucumber Dill Dip (page 124).

2 tablespoons vegetable broth

1 (15-ounce) can chickpeas, rinsed and drained

¼ cup chopped onions

2 garlic cloves

2 tablespoons chopped fresh parsley

½ teaspoon ground cumin

¾ teaspoon salt

¼ teaspoon black pepper

¼ cup garbanzo bean flour

Pita bread, for serving

Shredded lettuce, for serving

1 recipe *Cucumber Dill Dip* (page 124), for serving

1. Preheat oven to 350°F. Line a baking sheet with parchment.

2. Add vegetable broth, chickpeas, onions, garlic cloves, parsley, cumin, salt, and black pepper to a food processor. Blend until mixture begins to hold together.

3. Add mixture to a bowl and stir in garbanzo bean flour.

4. Form 12 small balls. Place on lined baking sheet. Bake for 20 minutes.

5. Serve on pita bread with shredded lettuce and cucumber dill dip.

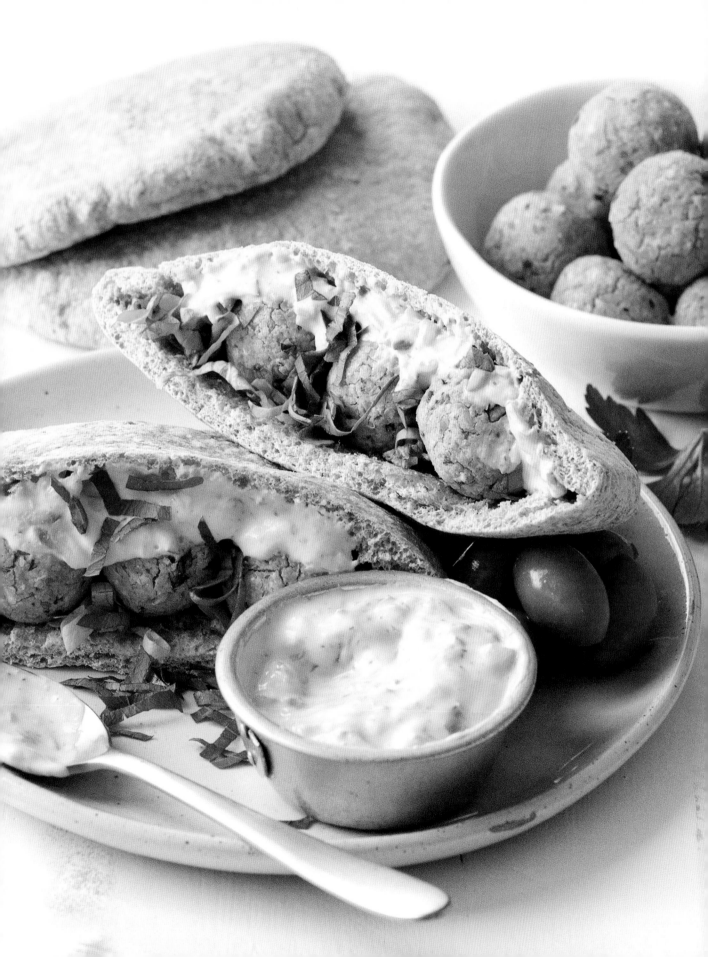

BLACK BEAN CHIPOTLE BURGERS

MAKES 6 BURGERS

Whenever I make Golden Cheese Sauce (page 171), I always double it, just to make these burgers. And if I have leftover burgers, I freeze them, placing each burger in a separate plastic bag so that I can reheat them one at a time. In doing this, I'm also preventing the burgers from sticking together. Serve the burgers with your favorite toppings; I like avocado, sprouts, and Chipotle Sauce (page 185).

¾–1 cup *Golden Cheese Sauce* (page 171), refrigerated for at least 2 hours

¼ cup finely chopped onions

½ cup cooked or canned black beans

½ cup corn

½ red bell pepper, finely diced

½ cup bread crumbs

1 tablespoon chopped fresh cilantro

½ teaspoon chipotle chile powder

¼ teaspoon salt

Sliced avocado, for serving

Sprouts, for serving

1 recipe *Chipotle Sauce* (page 185), for serving

1. Preheat oven to 350°F. Line a baking sheet with parchment.

2. Stir together ¾ cup chilled cheese sauce, onions, black beans, corn, bell pepper, bread crumbs, cilantro, chipotle powder, and salt. If the mixture is not holding together, add up to ¼ cup additional cheese sauce.

3. Form six ½-inch-thick patties. Place on lined baking sheet.

4. Bake for 35–40 minutes, flipping burgers after 20 minutes.

5. Top with avocado, sprouts, and chipotle sauce.

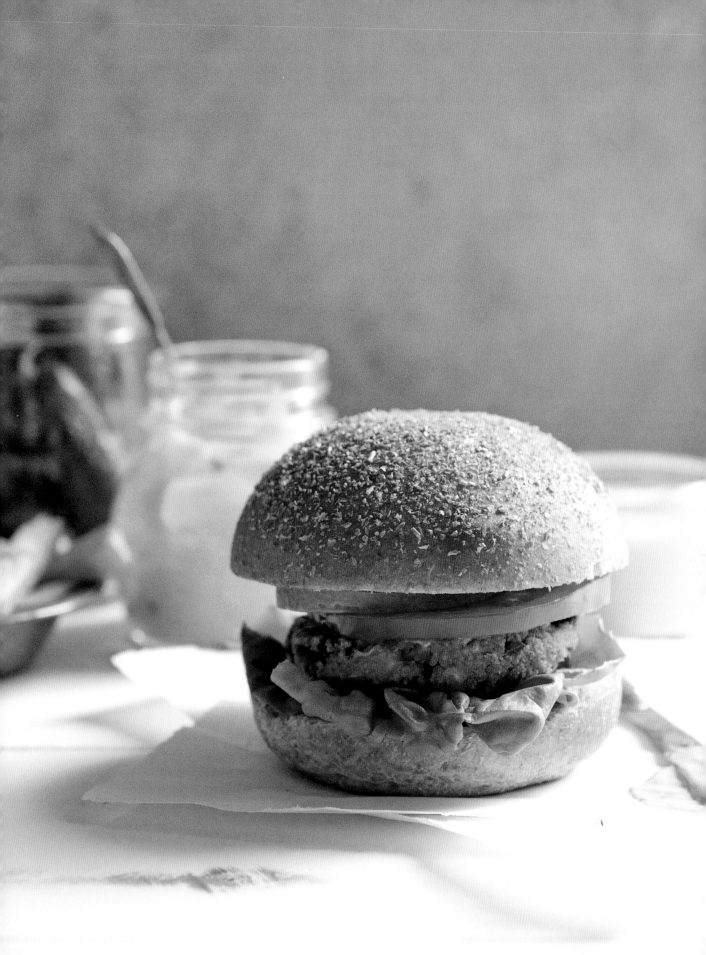

LENTIL COLLARD WRAPS WITH SALSA

MAKES 4 WRAPS

Collard leaves make a great substitute for breads and tortillas. They just need a quick blanch in boiling water to soften them. To assemble the wraps, pile all the ingredients in the middle of each leaf and then fold over as you would a burrito.

6 collard leaves
¾ cup brown rice
⅔ cup finely chopped onion
2 garlic cloves, minced
1¾ cups vegetable broth, divided
⅔ cup dried lentils, rinsed
1 teaspoon chili powder
½ teaspoon ground cumin
¼ teaspoon paprika
¼ teaspoon dried oregano
½ teaspoon salt, plus more to taste
Hot sauce, to taste
⅔ cup *Roasted Tomato Salsa* (page 121)
1 cup *Guacamole* (page 121)

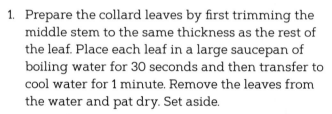

1. Prepare the collard leaves by first trimming the middle stem to the same thickness as the rest of the leaf. Place each leaf in a large saucepan of boiling water for 30 seconds and then transfer to cool water for 1 minute. Remove the leaves from the water and pat dry. Set aside.

2. Cook brown rice according to package directions. Set aside.

3. In a medium-size saucepan, sauté onion and garlic in 2 tablespoons of vegetable broth over medium-high heat for about 3 minutes, or until onion browns.

4. Add lentils, chili powder, cumin, paprika, oregano, salt, and hot sauce; cook and stir for 1 minute.

5. Add remaining vegetable broth and bring to a boil. Reduce heat to low, cover, and simmer until lentils are tender, 25–30 minutes.

6. Uncover and continue cooking until mixture is slightly thickened, 6–8 minutes. Stir in salsa.

7. Prepare the collard wraps by first spooning 2–3 tablespoons of rice on top of each leaf. Then spoon about 2–3 tablespoons lentil mixture on top of the rice, and finish by adding 2 heaping tablespoons guacamole.

8. Fold the collard leaf like a burrito, by first folding the bottom up, then the sides in. Enjoy!

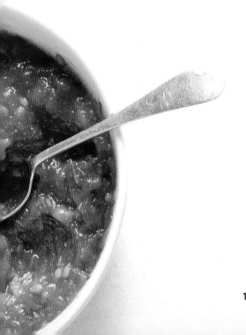

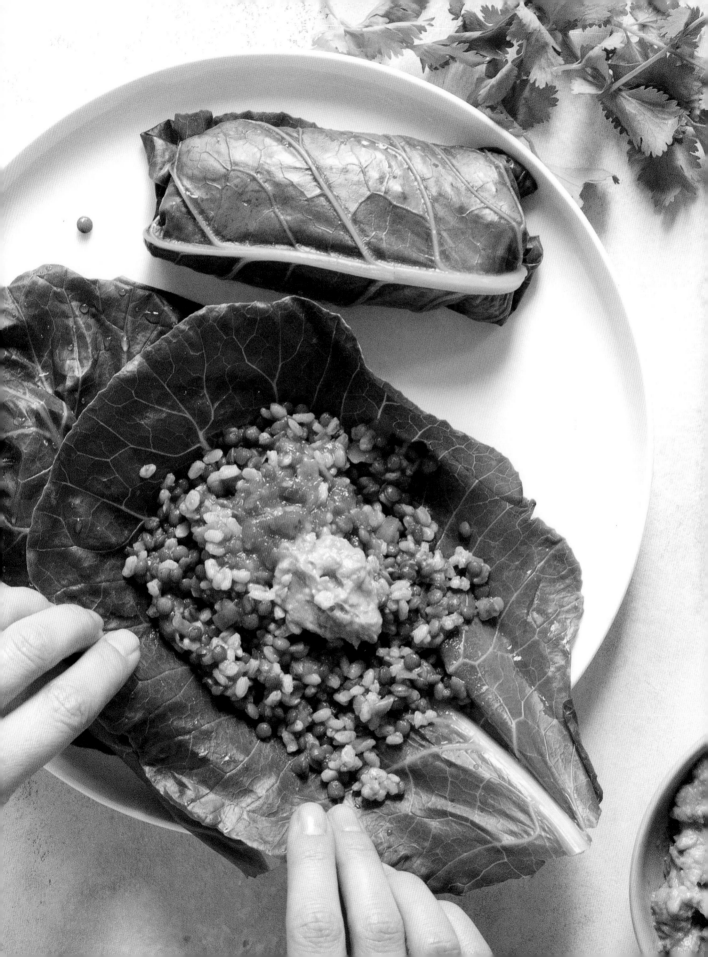

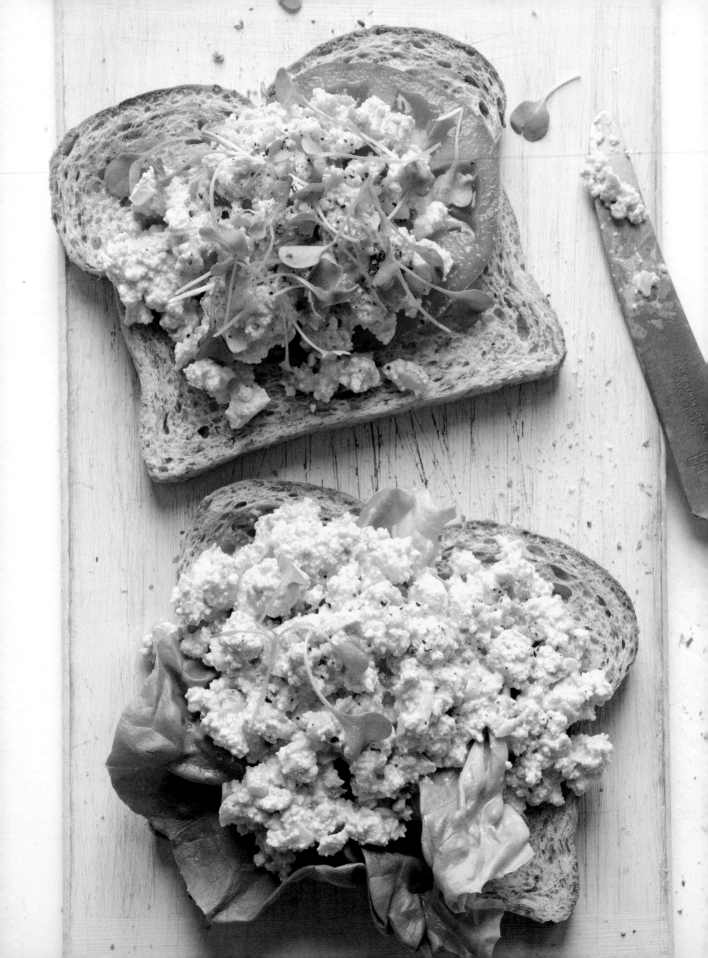

EGG(LESS) SALAD SANDWICH

MAKES 4 SANDWICHES

This vegetarian classic is one of the first sandwich spreads I learned to make. It's great in a wrap, in a pita pocket, or even on a baked potato. If serving in a wrap or pita pocket, stuff it with lettuce and tomatoes, then serve with Coconut Corn Chowder (page 134) or Quick Three-Bean Soup (page 148).

1 (12-ounce) package extra-firm tofu, drained and mashed

¼ cup *Golden Garden Mayonnaise* (page 184)

¼ cup diced dill pickles

¼ cup finely diced red onions

1 celery stalk, diced

1 medium carrot, finely grated

2 tablespoons rice vinegar

1 teaspoon ground mustard

½ teaspoon ground turmeric

½ teaspoon sea salt

8 slices whole wheat bread, for serving

Lettuce leaves, for serving

Tomato slices, for serving

1. Combine tofu, mayonnaise, pickles, onions, celery, carrot, vinegar, mustard, turmeric, and salt in a large mixing bowl. Mix thoroughly.

2. Spread on whole wheat bread and top with lettuce and tomato slices.

GRANOLA FRUIT WRAPS

MAKES 4 WRAPS

We first had these wraps on a hiking trip in Park City, Utah. My sons loved them! They were 9 and 10 at the time, and these wraps soon became a popular school lunch option. The fresh fruit is a great replacement for jam, and the granola is perfect with the peanut butter.

Natural peanut butter

4 large whole wheat tortillas, warmed

Nature's Granola (page 74)

Halved grapes or fresh blueberries

Diced apples

1. Spread peanut butter down the middle of each tortilla. Do not cover the entire tortilla.

2. Place two handfuls of granola on top of the peanut butter.

3. Place grapes and apples on top of granola.

4. Fold the tortilla, first from the bottom and then from the sides, like a burrito.

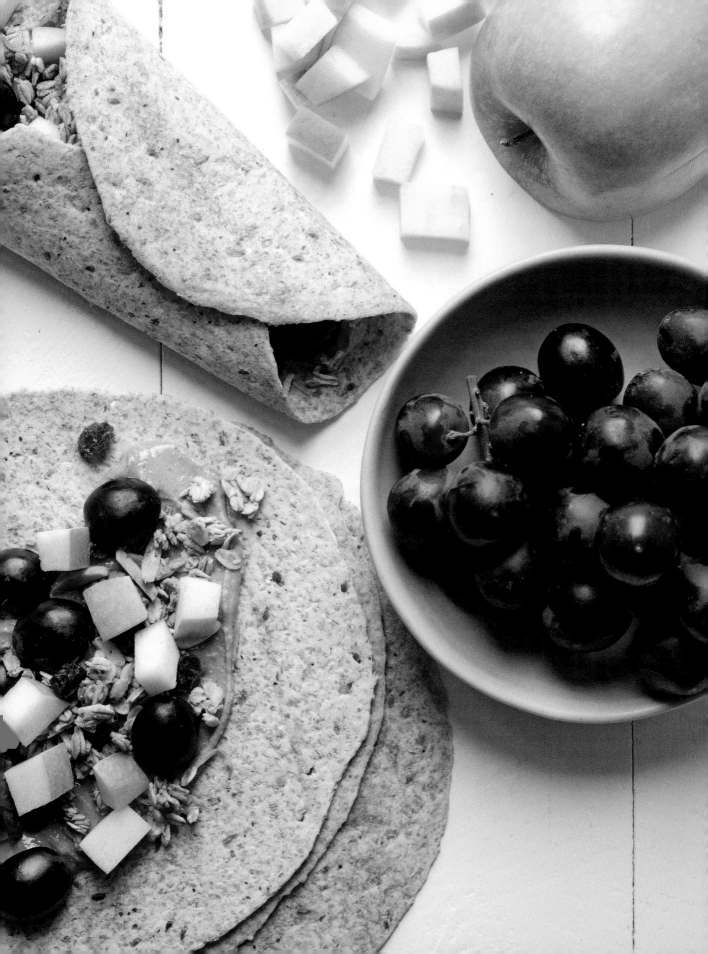

HAPPY TIME PORTOBELLOS

MAKES 4 SANDWICHES

You can't go wrong with a roasted portobello sandwich. I have one of these at least once a week. They're simple and tasty and can be topped with your favorite choice of sandwich spreads (pages 184–185) and fresh vegetables. I especially like spinach and Aioli Sauce (page 185).

4 large portobello mushroom caps

Salt and black pepper, to taste

4 large sandwiches buns,
   for serving

1 large tomato, sliced, for serving

1 medium red onion, thinly sliced,
   for serving

Spinach leaves, for serving

1 recipe *Aioli Sauce* (page 185),
   for serving

1. Preheat oven to 450°F. Line a baking sheet with parchment.

2. Sprinkle the mushroom caps with salt and black pepper, then place, stem-side down, on lined baking sheet.

3. Roast until tender, 18–20 minutes.

4. Assemble the burgers on the buns with tomato and onion slices, spinach, and aioli sauce.

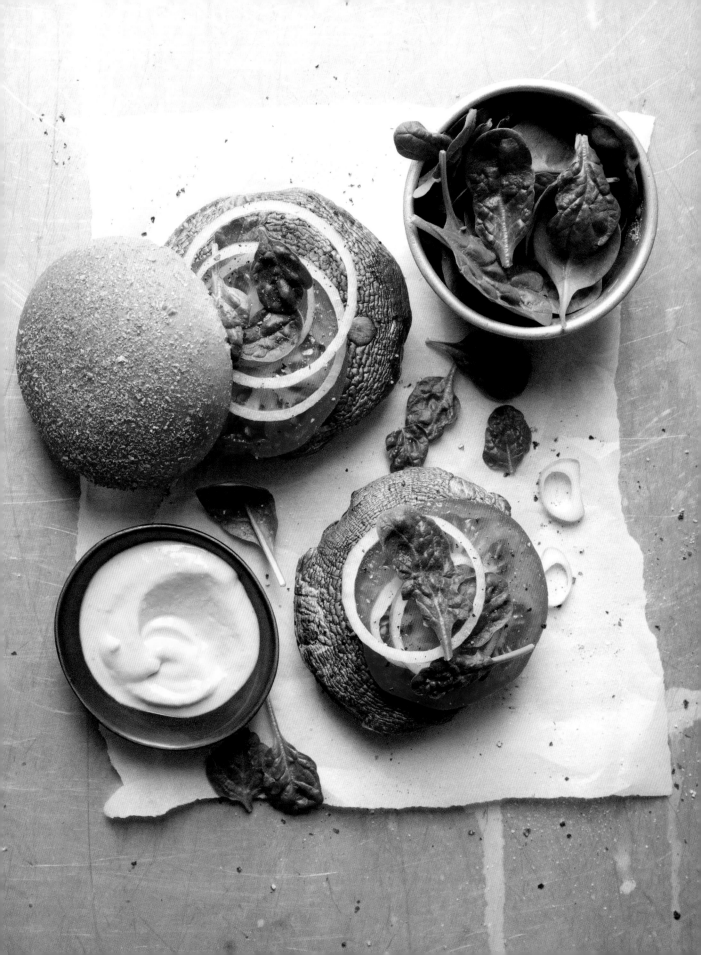

HUMMUS WRAPS

Hummus is a vegetarian classic. It's simple to make and can be tweaked in many different ways. It can be served with raw vegetables, on pitas, in wraps, or with your favorite bread. It can be topped with roasted vegetables, shredded lettuce, carrots, tomatoes, cucumbers, spinach, sautéed mushrooms— just about anything! My favorite is roasted red bell pepper hummus served in a pita, topped with roasted zucchini, sautéed mushrooms, and shredded lettuce.

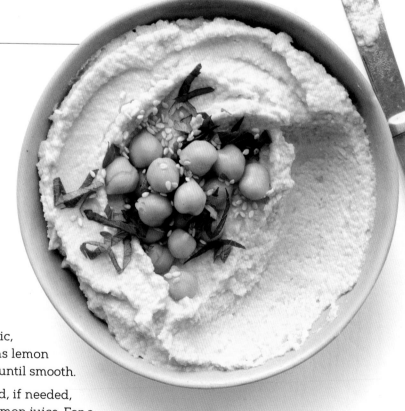

TRADITIONAL HUMMUS

MAKES 6 WRAPS

½ cup water
1 (15-ounce) can chickpeas, rinsed and drained
2 garlic cloves
½ cup sesame seeds
2–3 tablespoons lemon juice
Sea salt and ground cumin, to taste

1. Combine water, chickpeas, garlic, sesame seeds, and 2 tablespoons lemon juice in a food processor. Blend until smooth.

2. Season with salt and cumin and, if needed, up to 1 tablespoon additional lemon juice. For a creamier hummus, add more water.

ROASTED RED BELL PEPPER HUMMUS

To this same recipe, blend in ½ cup roasted red bell peppers.

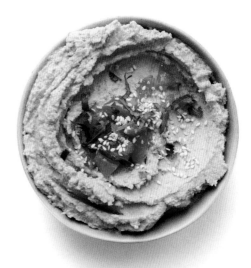

SUN-DRIED TOMATO HUMMUS WITH CAYENNE PEPPER

To this same recipe, blend in ½ cup sun-dried tomatoes and ⅛ teaspoon cayenne pepper.

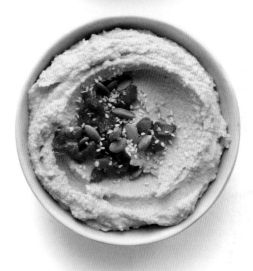

AVOCADO HUMMUS

To this same recipe, blend in flesh of 1 avocado and 1 tablespoon fresh cilantro.

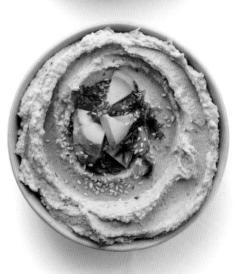

OCEAN CHICKPEA SANDWICHES

MAKES 6 SANDWICHES

Thirty years ago, tuna fish was one of my favorite sandwiches. Then I stopped eating tuna and found this recipe. To give it a fishy flavor, I use kelp powder; if I don't have any on hand, I use crumbled sushi wraps. However, I also enjoy it with just the smashed chickpeas, vegan mayonnaise, mustard, vinegar, dill pickles, celery, and onions.

1 (15-ounce) can chickpeas, rinsed and drained

5 tablespoons *Golden Garden Mayonnaise* (page 184)

1 tablespoon mustard

¼ cup diced dill pickles

¼ cup finely diced onions

1 celery stalk, diced

2 tablespoons rice vinegar

½ teaspoon kelp powder

Sea salt and black pepper, to taste

12 slices whole wheat bread, for serving

Lettuce leaves, for serving

Tomato slices, for serving

1. Place chickpeas in food processor and pulse 2–3 times; do not puree.

2. Transfer to a bowl. Add mayonnaise, mustard, pickles, onions, celery, rice vinegar, kelp powder, salt, and black pepper. Mix thoroughly.

3. Spread on whole wheat bread and top with lettuce and tomato slices.

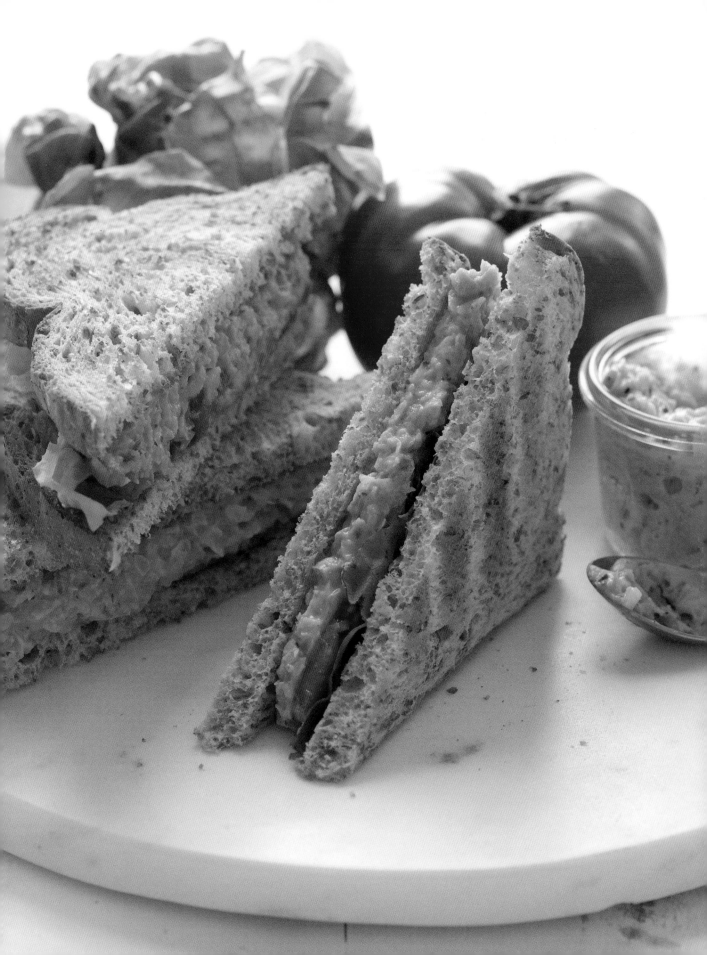

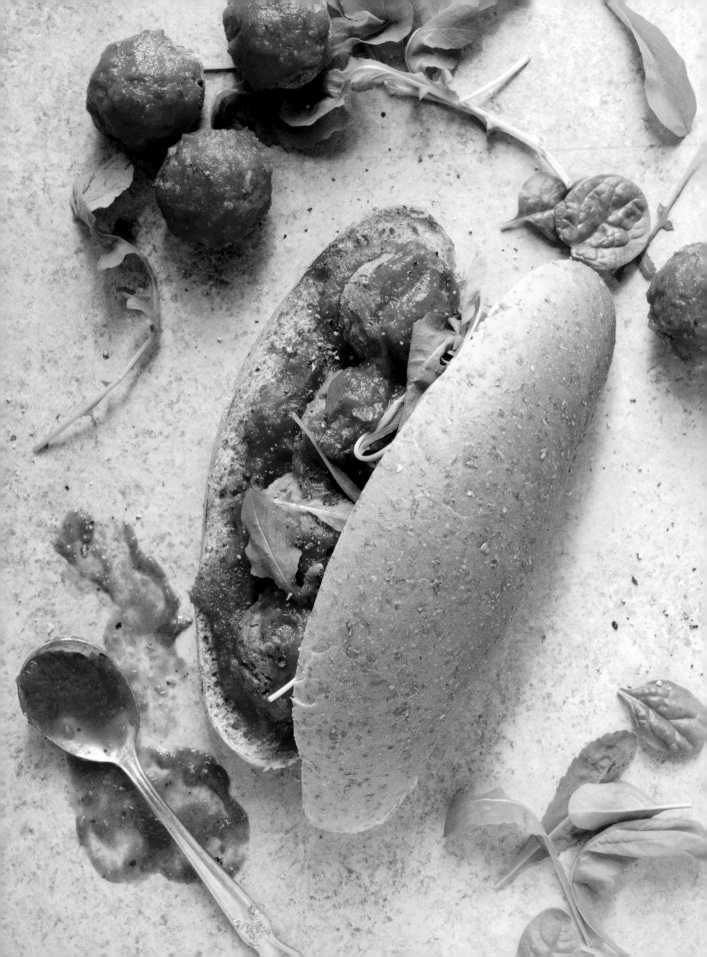

PECAN BALL SUBS

MAKES 4 SUBS

My mother's first "meatless" meatballs were pecan balls, served with spaghetti and marinara sauce. On the rare occasion when we had leftovers, she served them on sub rolls. When I make this recipe, I double it, freezing the leftovers for future subs.

—   —

½ cup pecans

1 (14-ounce) package extra-firm tofu

2 tablespoons reduced-sodium soy sauce

1 teaspoon dried thyme

½ teaspoon dried tarragon

½ teaspoon salt

½ cup chopped onions

½ cup chopped carrots

1 cup rolled oats

1 cup cooked brown rice

1 tablespoon flaxseed meal

4 whole wheat sub rolls

1 recipe *Favorite Marinara Sauce* (page 221)

1. Preheat oven to 350°F. Line a baking sheet with parchment.

2. In food processor, pulse pecans until fully ground. Transfer to mixing bowl.

3. Drain tofu and squeeze out all excess liquid. Pulse tofu, soy sauce, thyme, tarragon, salt, onions, and carrots in food processor until a ball forms. Add to pecan mixture.

4. Stir in oats, rice, and flaxseed meal.

5. Roll into balls, 2 inches in diameter, and place on lined baking sheet.

6. Bake for 45 minutes, turning over at 25 minutes.

7. Place pecan balls on sub rolls and top with marinara sauce.

ROASTED VEGGIE SUBS

MAKES 4 SUBS

Choose a roasted vegetable: eggplant, zucchini, or yellow squash. Top with tomatoes, green bell peppers, romaine lettuce, red onions, and Kalamata olives. Then add your favorite sandwich spread (pages 184–185) and enjoy!

1 eggplant, zucchini, or
  yellow squash

Dried oregano, salt, and black
  pepper, to taste

4 whole grain sub buns

1 large tomato, sliced

4 large lettuce or spinach leaves

¼ red onion, sliced

Sliced Kalamata olives

Savory Sandwich Spreads
  (pages 184–185)

1. Preheat oven to 400°F.

2. Slice eggplant, zucchini, or yellow squash. Spread out on a baking sheet. Season with oregano, salt, and black pepper. Bake for 10 minutes, turning at 5 minutes.

3. Assemble subs on buns with roasted veggies, tomatoes, lettuce or spinach, onions, olives, and sandwich spread.

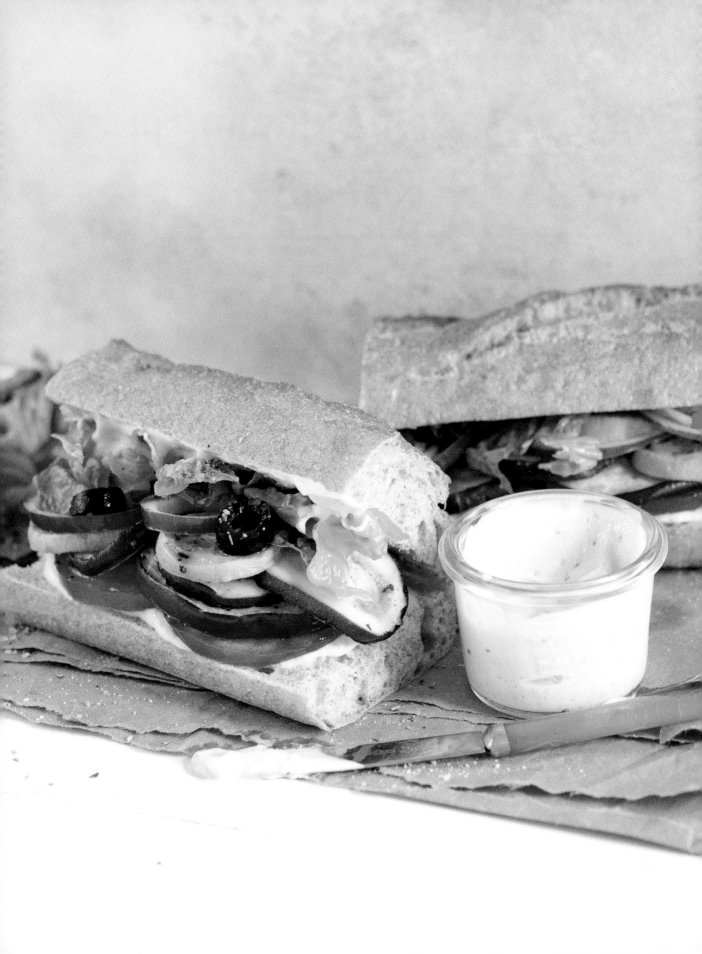

SAVORY SANDWICH SPREADS

It's always nice to have a jar of homemade plant-based mayonnaise in your refrigerator. I sometimes tweak the flavor of this spread by merely adding chipotle chile powder or minced garlic cloves and roasted red bell peppers. I use these spreads often—with burgers, subs, Egg(less) Salad Sandwiches (page 169), Ocean Chickpea Sandwiches (page 178), and salads.

GOLDEN GARDEN MAYONNAISE

MAKES 1 CUP

6 ounces soft silken tofu

¼ cup raw cashews

2 tablespoons lemon juice, plus more to taste

¼ teaspoon sea salt, plus more to taste

½ teaspoon Dijon mustard

1. Blend all ingredients in a food processor until smooth. Taste and add more salt and/or lemon juice if needed.

2. Store in an airtight container in the refrigerator.

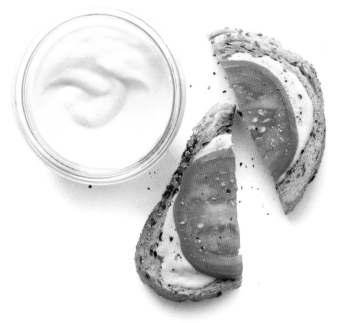

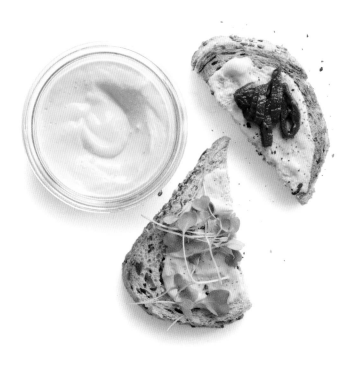

AIOLI SAUCE

MAKES 1 CUP

2 garlic cloves
1 small red bell pepper, cut in half and
  seeded
1 recipe *Golden Garden Mayonnaise*
  (page 184)

1. Preheat oven to 400°F.

2. Wrap garlic cloves and red pepper
   halves in aluminum foil and place on
   a baking sheet. Roast for 25 minutes.

3. Transfer roasted garlic and red bell
   pepper to a food processor. Add
   mayonnaise and blend until smooth.

4. Store in an airtight container in
   the refrigerator.

CHIPOTLE SAUCE

MAKES 1 CUP

1 recipe *Golden Garden Mayonnaise*
  (page 184)
1 teaspoon chipotle chile powder

1. Blend all ingredients in a food
   processor until smooth.

2. Store in an airtight container in
   the refrigerator.

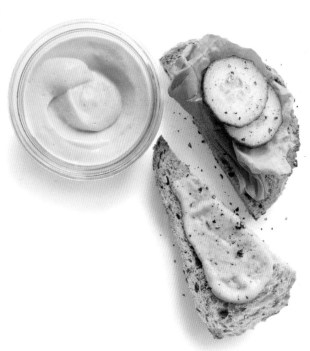

TACO BAR— YOUR CHOICE

When serving tacos, burritos, and tostados, I always prepare a small buffet with bowls of salsa, guacamole, shredded lettuce or spinach, refried beans, plain brown rice or Caribbean Moro (page 256), onions, bell peppers, tomatoes, roasted vegetables, baked sweet potatoes, sautéed mushrooms, Tomatillo Sauce (page 120), Golden Cheese Sauce (page 171), grated cabbage, black beans—you name it!

TOMATILLO TACKLE

MAKES 4 SERVINGS

½ cup grated cabbage

½ cup *Tomatillo Sauce* (page 120)

1 (15-ounce) can pinto beans, rinsed, drained, and blended until smooth (or vegan refried beans)

8 small tortillas, warmed

1 recipe *Golden Cheese Sauce* (page 171)

1 avocado, diced

1. In a small bowl, mix together cabbage and tomatillo sauce.

2. Heat pureed pinto beans in a skillet over medium heat for 3–4 minutes.

3. Spread 2–3 tablespoons beans on each tortilla. Top with cabbage mixture, cheese sauce, and avocado.

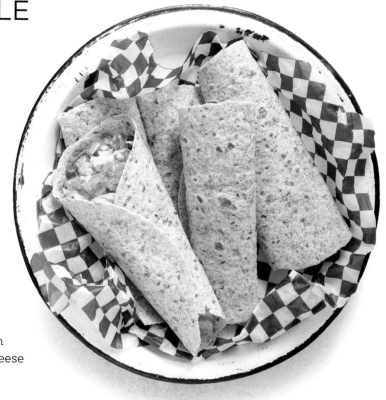

MUSHROOM, SPINACH, BLACK BEAN, AND GUACAMOLE COMBO

MAKES 4 SERVINGS

¼ cup sliced onions

2 tablespoons vegetable broth

2 cups sliced mushrooms

½ teaspoon chili powder

½ teaspoon ground cumin

⅛ teaspoon salt

1 (15-ounce) can black beans, rinsed, drained, and blended until smooth (or vegan refried beans)

8 small tortillas, warmed

¼ cup *Guacamole* (page 121)

½ cup baby spinach leaves

1. In a small saucepan, sauté onions in vegetable broth. Add mushrooms, chili powder, cumin, and salt. Cook until browned.

2. Heat pureed beans in skillet over medium heat for 3–4 minutes.

3. Spread 2–3 tablespoons beans on each tortilla and top with mushroom mixture, guacamole, and spinach.

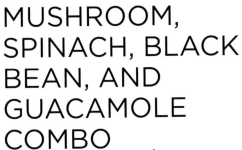

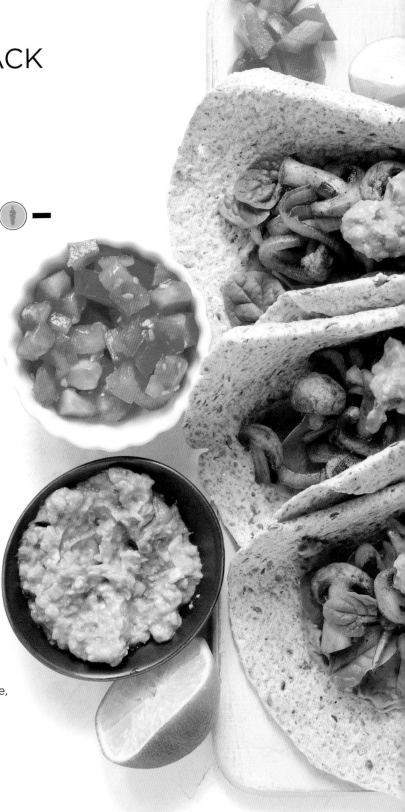

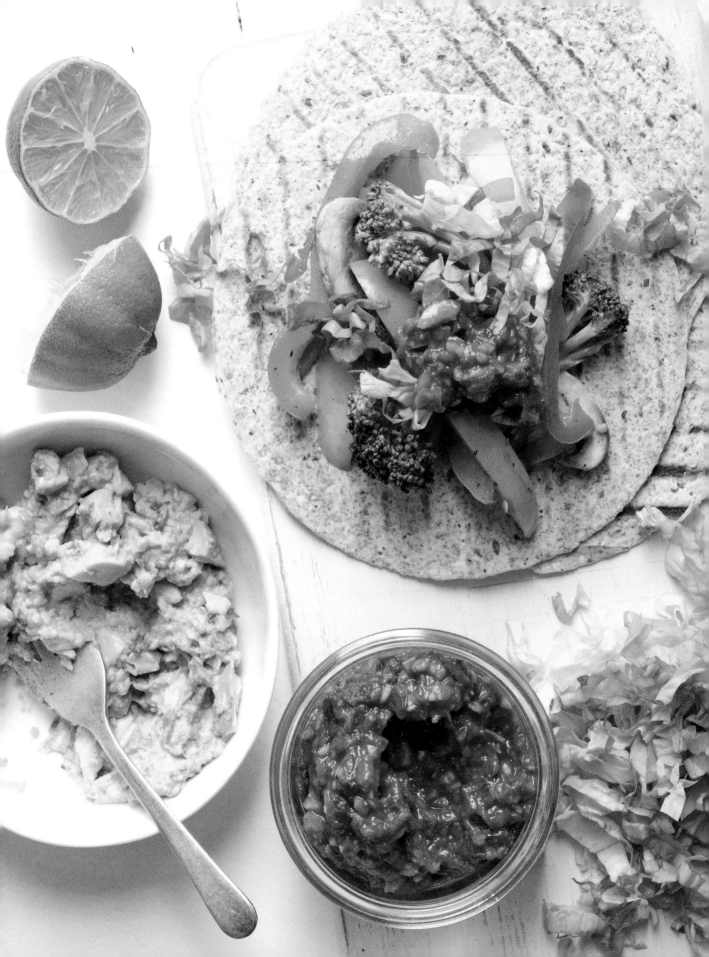

VEGGIE FAJITAS

MAKES 4 FAJITAS

One summer I hosted a group of seven artists for a two-week "Roots: Stories Through Murals" project. We would leave early in the morning and return late in the evening, famished, having had little or no lunch. This dish became our go-to meal. Within 10 minutes, we would have a large plate of fajitas on the table—large flour tortillas stuffed with lemon pepper vegetables, chopped lettuce, guacamole, and salsa. Yum!

2 garlic cloves, minced

½ onion, sliced

2 bell peppers (any color), seeded and sliced

4 tablespoons vegetable broth, divided

1 large carrot, sliced

1½ cups small broccoli florets

1 cup sliced mushrooms

1 lemon, cut in half

Lemon pepper seasoning and salt, to taste

4 large flour tortillas, warmed

1 cup chopped lettuce

1 recipe *Guacamole* (page 121)

1 recipe *Roasted Tomato Salsa* (page 121)

1. In a large skillet, sauté garlic, onion, and bell peppers in 2 tablespoons of vegetable broth over medium-high heat until veggies begin to brown.

2. Add remaining vegetable broth, carrot, broccoli, and mushrooms. Cover and cook over medium heat for 3–4 minutes. Squeeze the lemon halves over the veggies, then season with lemon pepper seasoning and salt.

3. To assemble the fajitas, place cooked veggies in the center of each tortilla, then top with chopped lettuce, guacamole, and salsa. Enjoy.

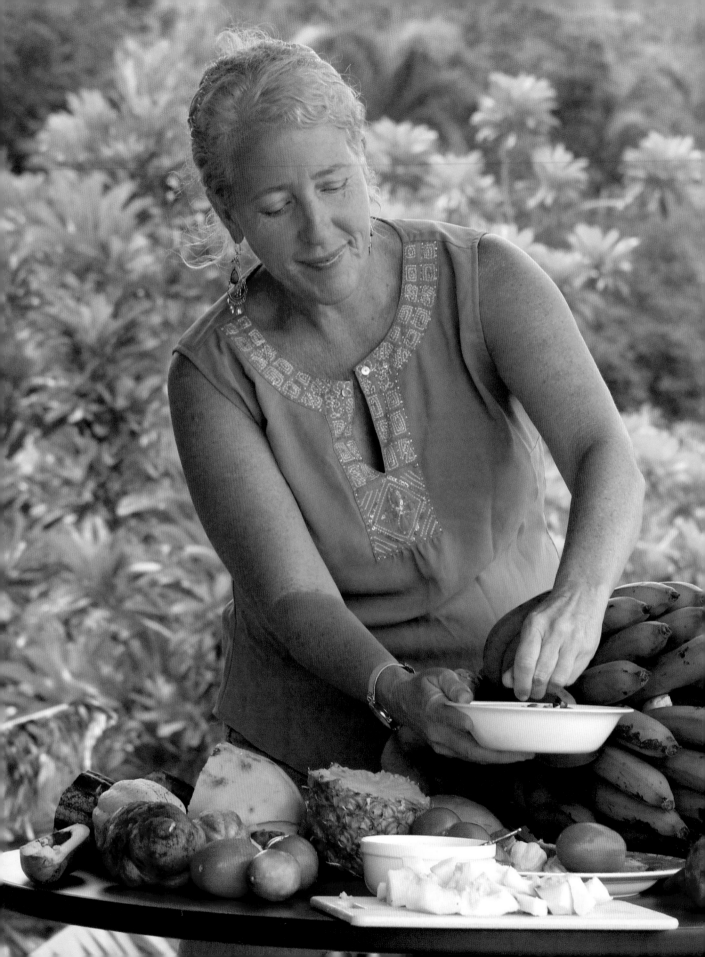

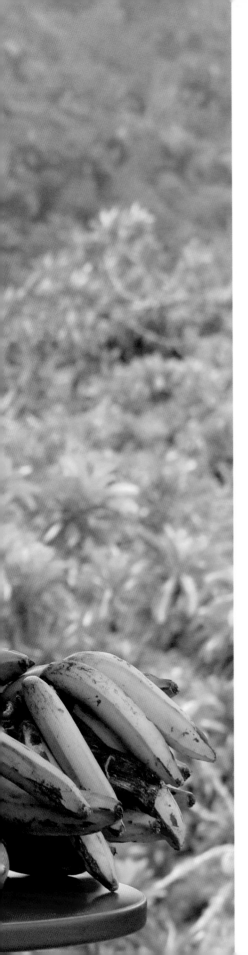

ENTRÉES

AFRICAN VEGETABLES

MAKES 6 SERVINGS

This rich, vibrantly flavored West African stew is often made with chicken. I've replaced the chicken with corn and zucchini, and it's one of our favorite meals. We especially like serving it with Simple Cabbage Slaw (page 100).

1 cup chopped onions

1 cup chopped green bell peppers

4 garlic cloves, minced

1 teaspoon grated fresh ginger

2 tablespoons vegetable broth

¼ teaspoon cayenne pepper

1 cup water

1 large sweet potato, peeled and cut into 1-inch cubes

1 medium zucchini, peeled and sliced

2 cups frozen chopped spinach

½ cup corn

1 (15-ounce) can diced tomatoes

2 tablespoons tomato paste

¼ cup natural peanut butter

Sea salt and black pepper, to taste

2 cups cooked brown rice, for serving

1. In a soup pot, sauté onions, bell peppers, garlic, and ginger in vegetable broth over medium-high heat until onions brown.

2. Reduce heat to medium. Add cayenne pepper and cook for 1–2 minutes longer.

3. Add water, sweet potato, zucchini, frozen spinach, corn, tomatoes, and tomato paste. Bring the mixture to a simmer, reduce heat, cover, and cook for 15 minutes, until sweet potato is easily pierced with a fork. If necessary, add more water.

4. Stir in peanut butter and season with salt and black pepper. Cover and cook for an additional 3–5 minutes.

5. Serve over cooked rice.

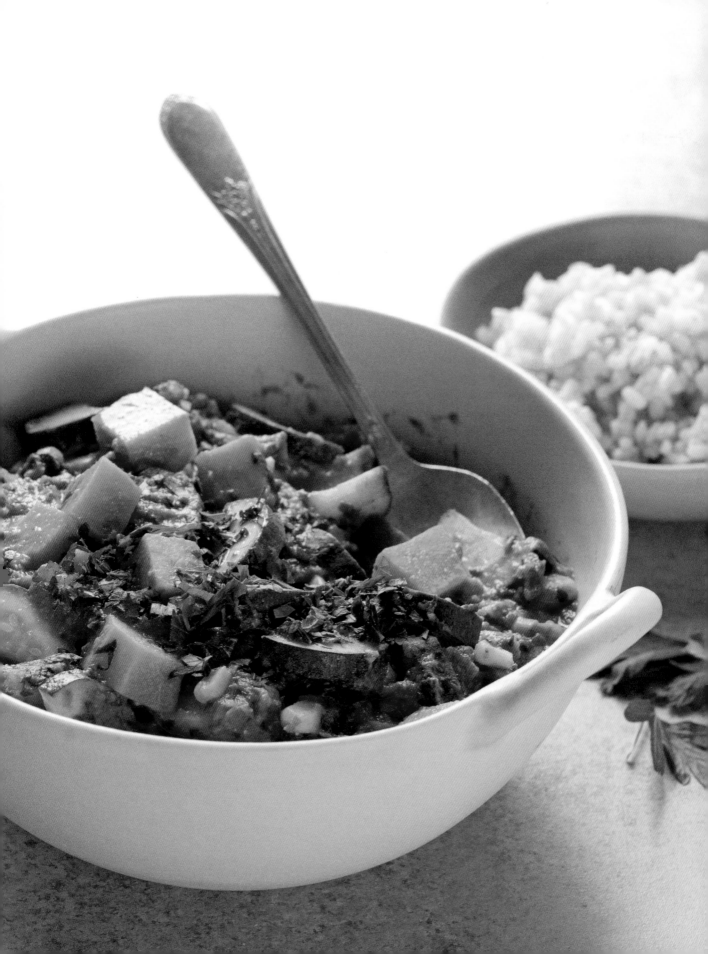

ASPARAGUS CRÊPES

MAKES 6 CRÊPES

My mother used to make this dish with melted cheese. When she didn't have asparagus, she would use green beans. However, asparagus was always our preferred choice. The lemon cashew sauce used in this recipe is a lot better than melted cheese, and it's great served with a fresh Kale Salad with Sweet Potatoes (page 112).

Crêpes

1 cup whole wheat pastry flour

⅛ teaspoon salt

2 egg replacers (2 tablespoons ground flaxseed meal mixed with 6 tablespoons water)

2 cups unsweetened nondairy milk (rice, soy, almond, etc.)

Sauce

6 ounces soft silken tofu

½ cup raw cashews

¾ teaspoon sea salt

¼ cup plus 2 tablespoons lemon juice

½ teaspoon Dijon mustard

2 tablespoons nutritional yeast

½ cup water

Pinch of red pepper flakes

Filling

3 garlic cloves, minced

3 cups bite-size asparagus pieces

2 tablespoons vegetable broth

2 tablespoons lemon juice

1 teaspoon onion powder

½ teaspoon sea salt

¼ teaspoon dried tarragon

1. Preheat oven to 350°F.

2. For the crêpes, in a large bowl, whisk flour, salt, egg replacers, and milk until batter is smooth. Add more milk if needed.

3. Heat a nonstick skillet over medium heat until hot. Pour about ¼ cup of batter evenly over bottom of pan. Tilt and rotate the skillet until batter is spread evenly. Cook the crêpe until it is fully cooked. If you try to flip it too soon, it will fold over on itself and stick to the bottom of the skillet. Shake the pan, and if the crêpe lifts, it is ready to flip. Cook the other side until brown. Repeat this process with the remaining batter.

4. If the batter thickens while making the crêpes, thin it with a little extra milk. Set the crêpes aside.

5. For the sauce, blend all ingredients in a food processor until smooth. Set aside.

6. For the filling, dry sauté the garlic. Add the asparagus, vegetable broth, lemon juice, onion powder, salt, and tarragon. Cover and cook over medium heat for 3–5 minutes, until asparagus becomes tender.

7. To assemble, place ½ cup of asparagus in the center of each crêpe. Roll up and place in a large nonstick baking dish. Continue until all crêpes are filled.

8. Spread sauce on top of crêpes, cover with aluminum foil, and bake for 20 minutes. Serve immediately.

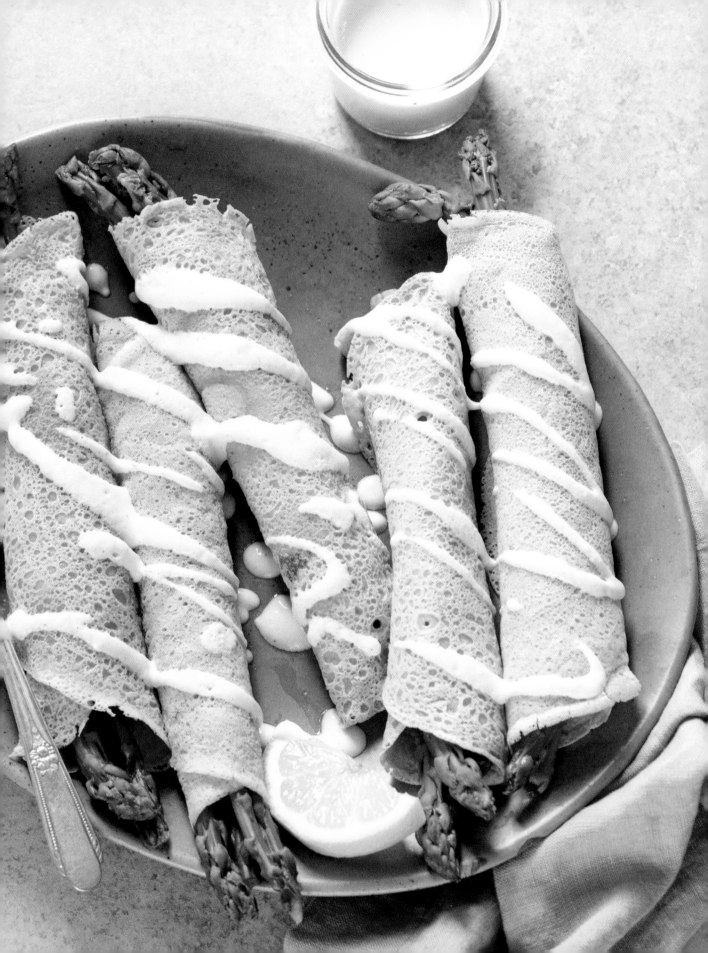

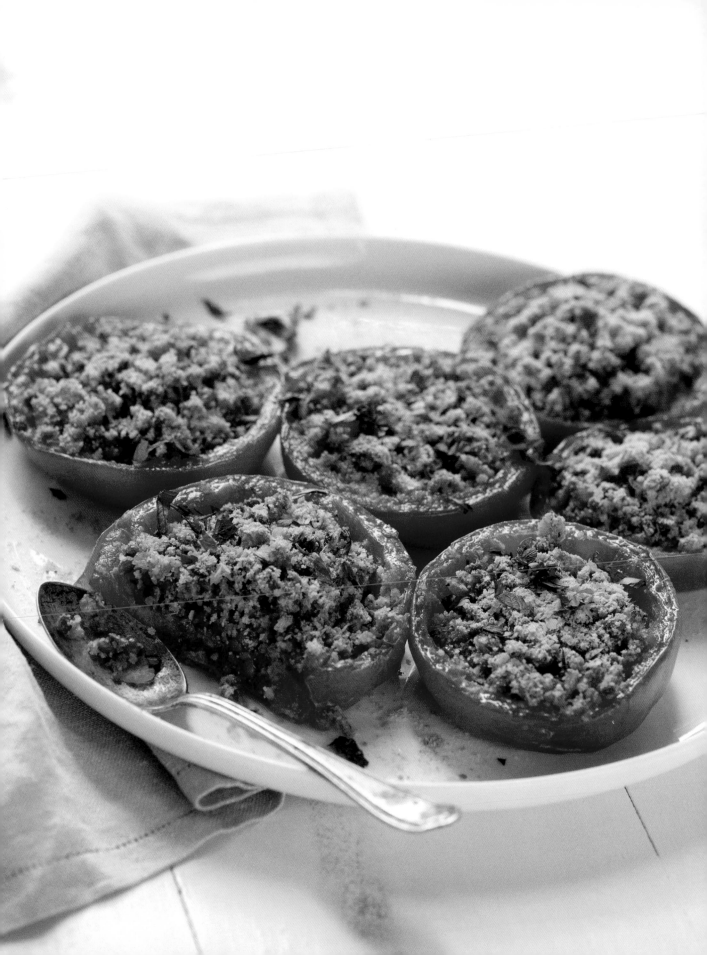

BAKED TOMATOES WITH LENTILS

MAKES 3-4 SERVINGS

Compared to other dried beans, lentils cook quickly and easily. They work well in stuffings and loaves. I especially like them with tomatoes, onions, garlic, and oregano. To make a heartier stuffing, I like to use whole wheat bread crumbs.

3 large, firm tomatoes
½ cup diced onions
3 garlic cloves, minced
2 tablespoons vegetable broth
2 teaspoons dried oregano
¾ teaspoon salt
⅛ teaspoon black pepper
1½ cups cooked lentils
½ cup whole wheat bread crumbs

1. Preheat oven to 350˚F.

2. Cut the tomatoes in half and scoop the insides into a bowl. Turn the tomato shells upside down to drain while preparing the stuffing.

3. In a nonstick skillet, sauté onions and garlic in vegetable broth over medium-high heat until onions brown.

4. Add oregano, salt, black pepper, and insides of the tomatoes. Cook for 2–3 minutes. Remove from heat.

5. Stir in lentils and bread crumbs.

6. Spoon the lentil mixture into the tomato shells and place in a small baking dish.

7. Bake, uncovered, for 20–25 minutes. Serve warm.

BLACK BEAN CAULIFLOWER BURRITOS

MAKES 4 SERVINGS

While living in Mississippi, we found a small Mexican restaurant that served soft tacos stuffed with mashed potatoes and spinach. My sons loved them. This is a spinoff of that dish. Instead of mashed potatoes, I use Creamed Cauliflower (page 254), and I add black beans. We sometimes serve this for breakfast, in place of our Savory Southwestern Burritos (page 80).

1 recipe *Creamed Cauliflower* (page 254)

4 large whole grain tortillas

1 cup cooked or canned black beans

1 cup chopped spinach

1 (15-ounce) jar salsa

1. Preheat oven to 375°F.

2. Spoon 3–4 tablespoons creamed cauliflower down the center of each tortilla. Top with 2 tablespoons black beans, then add some spinach and salsa.

3. Fold up the bottom of the burrito, then fold over both sides.

4. Place burritos, seam-side down, in a nonstick baking pan. Spread additional salsa across the top of the burritos.

5. Bake for 10 minutes. Serve immediately.

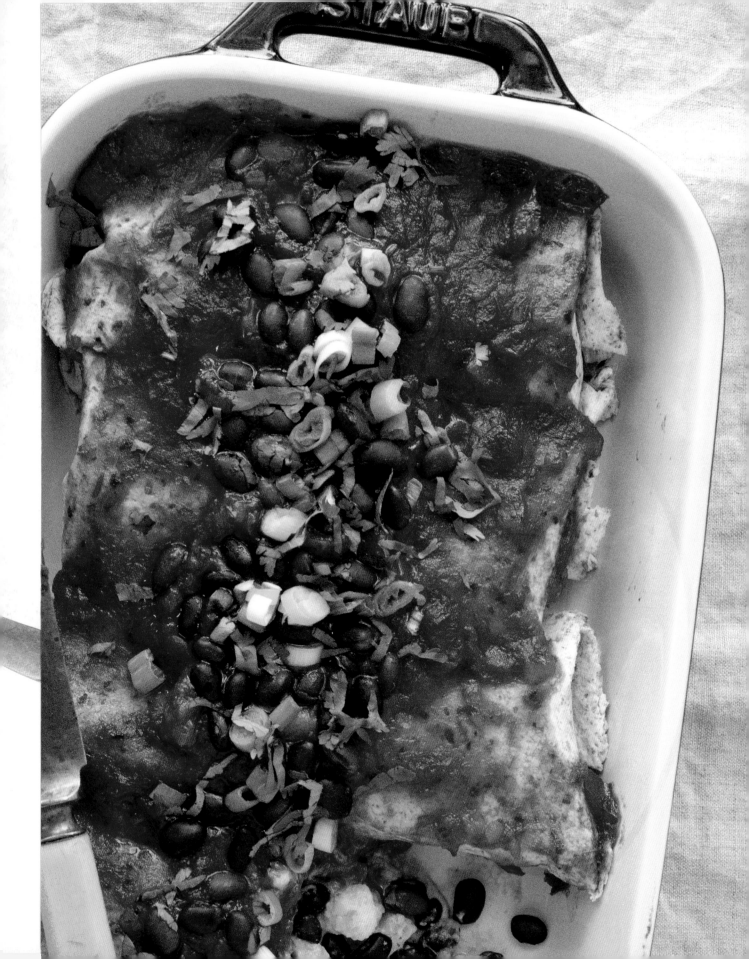

CARROT BAKE

MAKES 4–6 SERVINGS

This is a wonderful Thanksgiving dish, but it can be served at any time during the year. The first layer consists of a savory carrot stuffing, followed by mashed potatoes, then topped with mushroom gravy. It goes well with Cranberry Applesauce (page 262), Coconut Creamed Corn (page 261), and Broccoli Walnut Salad (page 96).

Carrot Stuffing

2½ cups grated carrots

½ cup diced onions

½ cup diced celery

½ cup vegetable broth

1 teaspoon dried thyme

½ teaspoon dried rosemary

½ teaspoon salt

¼ teaspoon black pepper

1 cup whole wheat bread crumbs

2 egg replacers (2 tablespoons ground flaxseed meal mixed with 6 tablespoons water)

Mashed Potatoes

3 medium potatoes, peeled and diced

2 tablespoons unsweetened nondairy milk (rice, soy, almond, etc.)

¼ teaspoon garlic powder

¼ teaspoon sea salt

Mushroom Gravy

2 tablespoons minced onion

1 tablespoon vegetable broth

1 cup chopped mushrooms

¼ teaspoon dried thyme

1 cup unsweetened nondairy milk (soy or almond)

1 tablespoon cornstarch

Salt and black pepper, to taste

1. Preheat oven to 350°F.

2. To make stuffing, in a medium-size saucepan, sauté carrots, onions, and celery in vegetable broth over medium-high heat until onions are soft. Remove from heat. Add thyme, rosemary, salt, black pepper, bread crumbs, and egg replacers. Mix well.

3. Spread mixture in a nonstick baking dish. Bake for 20 minutes, until top is slightly crisp.

4. Meanwhile, put potatoes in a large saucepan and cover with water. Bring water to a boil over medium-high heat and cook until potatoes are soft. Drain.

5. Blend potatoes, milk, garlic powder, and salt in a food processor. Spread on top of cooked carrot mixture.

6. To make gravy, in a medium saucepan, sauté onion in vegetable broth over medium heat until brown. Add mushrooms and thyme and cook for 2 minutes. Whisk together milk and cornstarch. Stir into mushroom mixture and cook until sauce thickens. Season with salt and black pepper.

7. Pour gravy over mashed potatoes and carrot stuffing and serve.

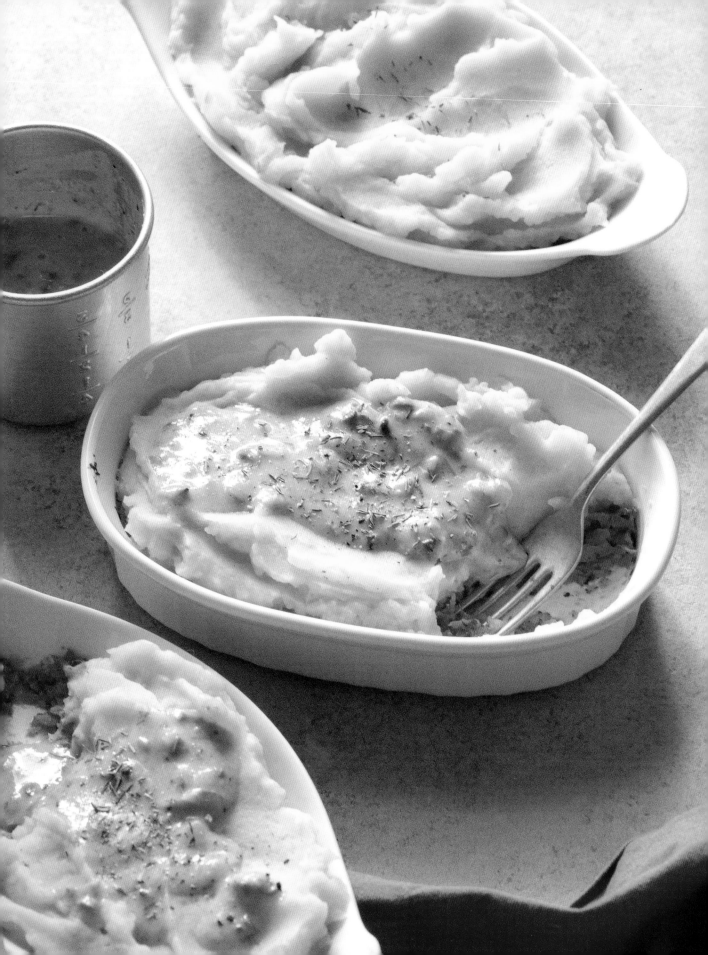

CREAMY CAULIFLOWER FETTUCCINE WITH BROCCOLI

MAKES 6 SERVINGS

Cauliflower can be prepared in many different ways: creamed (page 254), as a stand-in for rice (page 255), or as in this recipe, where I use cauliflower to make a creamy Alfredo sauce. When adding vegetables, make sure to steam them separately, then toss them in at the end.

3–4 cups small broccoli florets

3 cups cauliflower florets

1 cup cashews

1 cup unsweetened nondairy milk (soy or almond)

½ teaspoon lemon juice

¼ cup nutritional yeast

1 teaspoon garlic powder

½ teaspoon salt

¼ teaspoon black pepper

16 ounces fettuccine, cooked

1. Steam broccoli in a saucepan over boiling water until tender, about 5 minutes. It should be green and crunchy. Drain and set aside.

2. Put cauliflower in same saucepan, cover with water, and simmer for 5–7 minutes, until soft. Drain.

3. In a food processor, blend cauliflower, cashews, milk, lemon, nutritional yeast, garlic powder, salt, and black pepper until smooth.

4. Pour sauce over fettuccine, then fold in steamed broccoli. Serve warm.

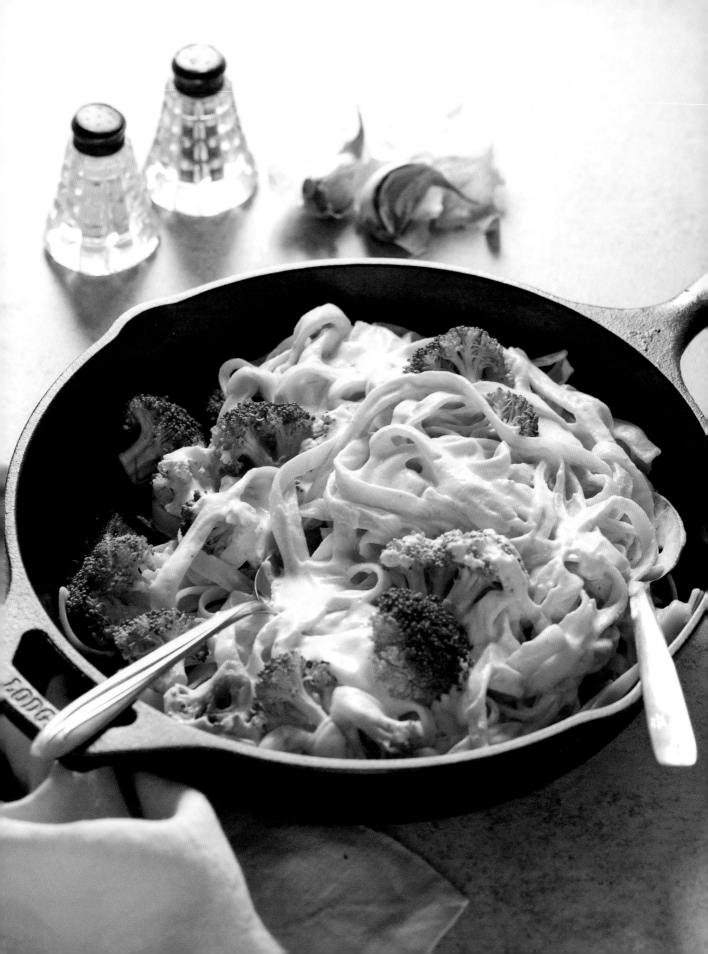

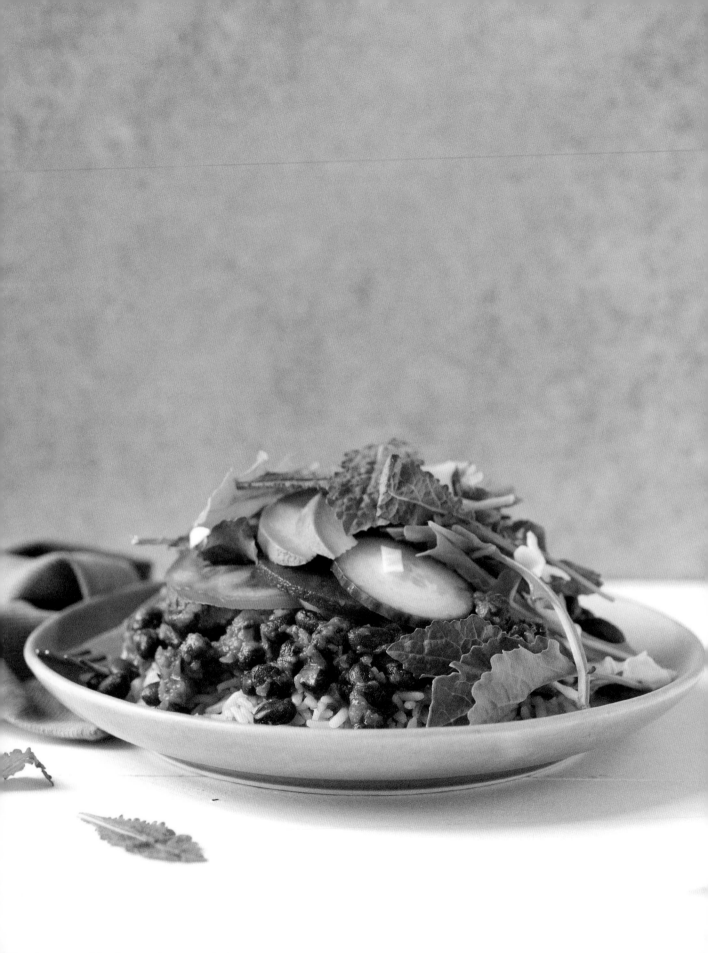

DOMINICAN RICE AND BEANS

MAKES 6–8 SERVINGS

My sons, now 24 and 23, were raised on a plant-based diet, and if you ask them what their favorite meal is, they both immediately respond Dominican Rice and Beans, topped with fresh salad. The secret to this meal is to top the rice and beans with fresh salad and avocados, then drizzle with lemon juice and/or rice vinegar.

Rice and Beans

¼ cup diced onions

4 garlic cloves, minced

½ cup chopped green bell peppers

¼ cup chopped fresh cilantro

2 tablespoons vegetable broth

2 cups water

2 (15-ounce) cans beans of your choice (pinto, black, red, etc.), rinsed and drained

½ cup grated butternut squash

1½ tablespoons tomato paste

1 teaspoon salt

4 cups cooked brown rice, for serving

Salad

2 cups sliced lettuce

2 cups sliced cabbage

¾ cup sliced cucumber

¾ cup sliced beets

1 tomato, sliced

1 large avocado, pitted and sliced

3 tablespoons rice vinegar

3 tablespoons water

¼ teaspoon salt, plus more to taste

1. In a large saucepan, sauté onions, garlic, bell peppers, and cilantro in vegetable broth over medium-high heat until onions brown.

2. Add water, beans, and squash. Bring to a low simmer and cook, uncovered, for 10 minutes.

3. While the beans are cooking, prepare the salad. In a large salad bowl, toss together all ingredients. Set aside.

4. Once the beans cook, add tomato paste and salt. Taste and add more salt if needed. Cook for 2–3 more minutes. Remove from heat.

5. Serve beans over rice and top with salad.

EGGPLANT "PARMESAN"

MAKES 4 SERVINGS

We have been preparing this simple dish for at least 25 years. You can serve the eggplant after removing it from the oven, but I like to go the extra step and bake it with our Favorite Marinara Sauce (page 221). I then serve it over pasta, with additional sauce if needed.

½ cup whole grain pastry flour

½–¾ cup unsweetened nondairy milk (rice, soy, almond, etc.)

1–2 cups Italian bread crumbs

1 large eggplant, peeled and sliced lengthwise ¼–½-inch thick

2 (28-ounce) jars marinara sauce or triple batch of *Favorite Marinara Sauce* (page 221)

10 ounces spaghetti, cooked

1. Preheat oven to 350°F. Line a baking sheet with parchment.

2. Place pastry flour in a shallow bowl, milk in a second shallow bowl, and bread crumbs in a third shallow bowl. Bread eggplant slices by first dipping each slice in the flour, then covering with milk, and then dredging in bread crumbs. You may need to add more flour, milk, or bread crumbs depending on the number of slices your eggplant yields.

3. Place breaded eggplant on lined baking sheet. Bake for 20 minutes, until brown, turning halfway through. Remove from oven, but keep oven on.

4. Spread ½ cup marinara sauce over bottom of a 3-quart baking dish. Layer with eggplant slices. Add another layer of marinara sauce. Top with remaining eggplant slices and cover with marinara sauce.

5. Cover with aluminum foil and bake for 30 minutes. Serve on top of spaghetti and have extra marinara sauce on hand, if needed.

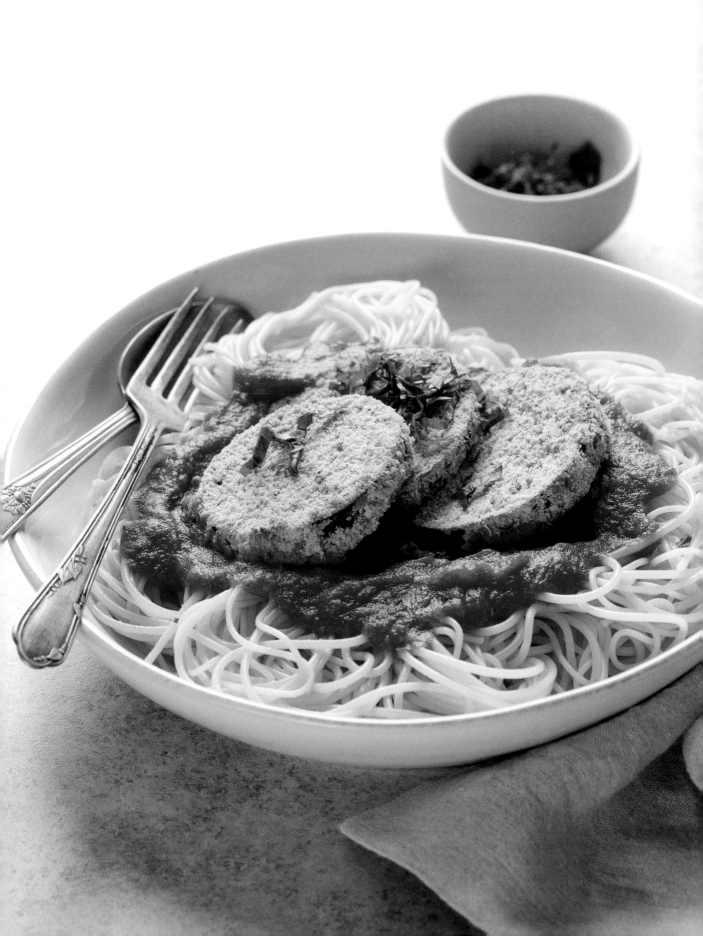

FAVORITE CHILI WITH PASTA

MAKES 6 SERVINGS

Super easy and tasty, this dish can be made in 10–15 minutes. While the pasta is cooking, I prepare the chili. I save time by using canned tomatoes, canned kidney beans, and frozen corn, but make sure to check the salt content for the canned tomatoes.

1 cup diced onions

4 garlic cloves, minced

1 tablespoon dried oregano

1 tablespoon chili powder

2 tablespoons vegetable broth

1 (15-ounce) can kidney beans, rinsed and drained

1 (15-ounce) can diced tomatoes with jalapeños

1 cup chopped green bell peppers

1 large carrot, grated

2 cups corn

1 teaspoon salt

8 ounces pasta, cooked

1. In a medium-size skillet, sauté onions, garlic, oregano, and chili powder in vegetable broth over medium-high heat until onions brown.

2. Add kidney beans, tomatoes, bell peppers, carrot, corn, and salt. Cover and cook over medium heat for 12–15 minutes.

3. Serve on top of cooked pasta.

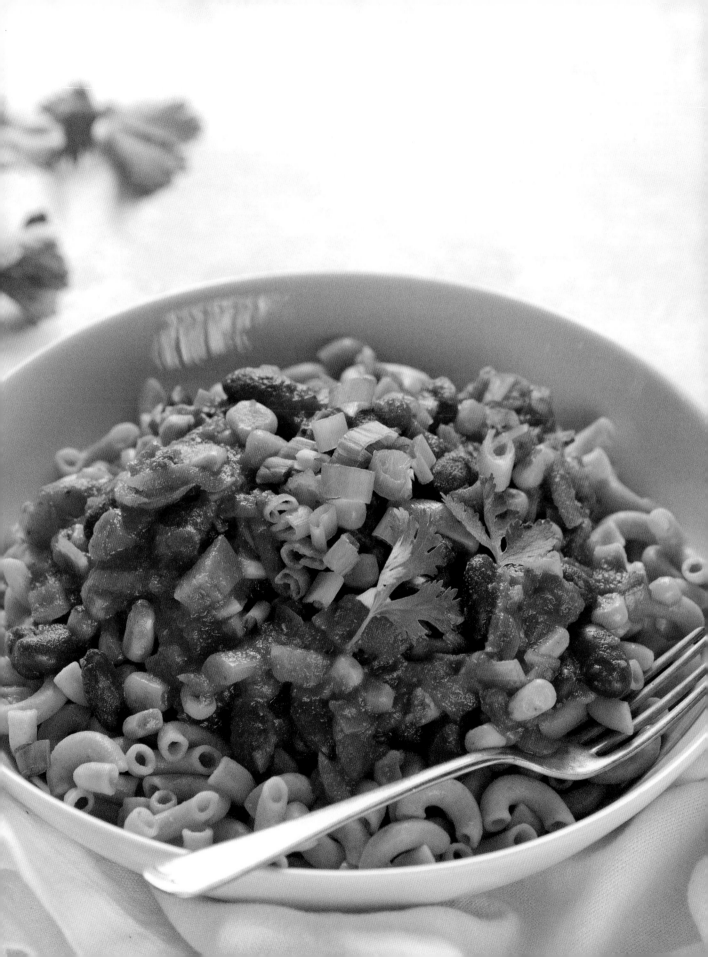

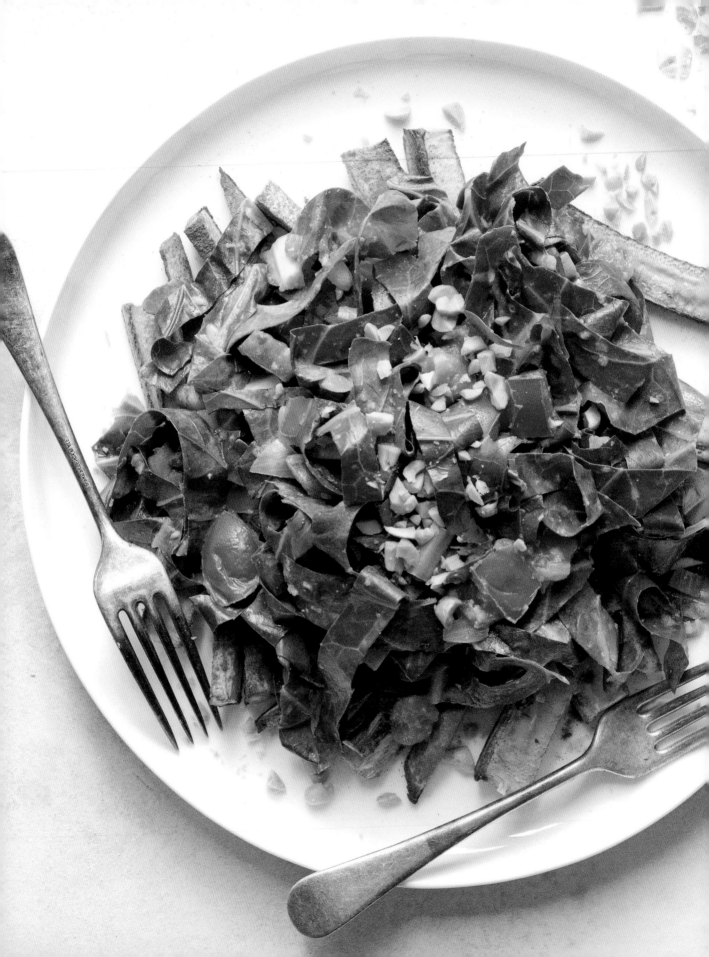

GIVE-ME-MORE PEANUT COLLARDS

MAKES 3-4 SERVINGS

I first had a dish similar to this on Mother's Day, ten years ago, when my sons treated me to dinner at an African restaurant. Later my younger son made a dish similar to this and kept telling me to try it. I did and I was hooked. But what makes this recipe so good is that I serve it on top of Plátanos Maduros (page 267).

½ cup diced onions

4 garlic cloves, minced

⅛ teaspoon red pepper flakes (optional)

4 tablespoons vegetable broth, divided

4 cups chopped collard greens

2 tomatoes, diced

2 tablespoons natural peanut butter mixed with ¼ cup vegetable broth

½ teaspoon lemon juice

Salt, to taste

½ cup crushed peanuts

1 recipe *Plátanos Maduros* (page 267), for serving

1. In a medium saucepan, sauté onions, garlic, and red pepper flakes (if using) in 2 tablespoons of vegetable broth over medium-high heat for 3–5 minutes, until onions brown.

2. Add remaining 2 tablespoons of vegetable broth, collard greens, and tomatoes. Cover and cook over medium heat for 3–5 minutes.

3. Add peanut butter mixture and lemon juice. Cook for 2–3 minutes.

4. Season with salt and add crushed peanuts.

5. Serve peanut collards on top of maduros.

LEAFY LENTILS

MAKES 4 SERVINGS

This dish is especially good with Greek Salad with Tofu "Feta" (page 111), Carrot Beet Slaw (page 101), or Simple Cabbage Slaw (page 100), but I also sometimes serve it with a simple salad of greens, cucumbers, tomatoes, and balsamic vinegar.

1 large onion, diced

6 garlic cloves, minced

3 cups vegetable broth, divided

1 cup uncooked brown lentils

1 (15-ounce) can diced tomatoes
  with jalapeños

3 tablespoons dried oregano

3 tablespoons tomato paste

2 cups chopped spinach

1 tablespoon balsamic vinegar

Salt and black pepper, to taste

4 cups cooked brown rice,
  for serving

1. In a large soup pot, sauté onions and garlic in 2 tablespoons of vegetable broth over medium-high heat until onions brown.

2. Add remaining vegetable broth, lentils, tomatoes, and oregano. Cover and simmer for 20 minutes, until lentils are tender but not mushy. Be careful not to overcook.

3. Stir in tomato paste and spinach. Cover and cook on low until spinach is wilted, 2–3 minutes. Remove from heat.

4. Add vinegar and season with salt and black pepper. Serve over brown rice.

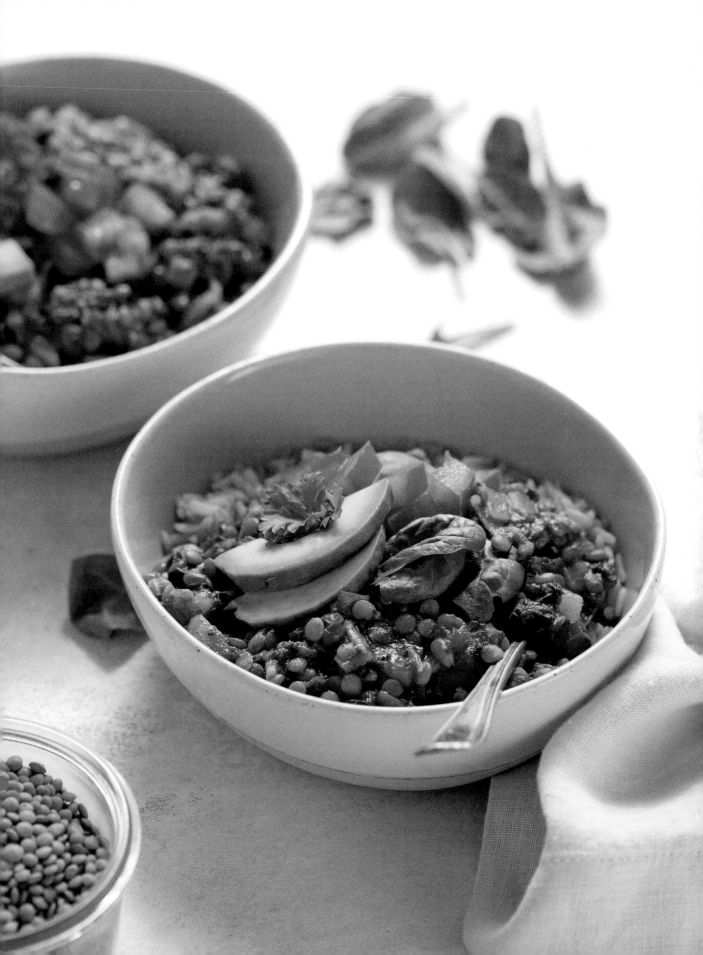

MACARONI SQUASH

MAKES 4 SERVINGS

There are many versions to this recipe, and it has always been my younger son's favorite dish. I like to use butternut squash, cashews, and a bit of nutritional yeast and miso. I have made it for my sons' meat-eating, cheese-loving friends, and they always gobble it up.

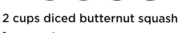

2 cups diced butternut squash

1 cup water

½ cup raw cashews

2 tablespoons nutritional yeast

2 tablespoons white miso

1 teaspoon lemon juice

1 tablespoon onion powder

1 teaspoon salt, plus more to taste

¼ teaspoon black pepper

1 pound macaroni, cooked

1. Preheat oven to 350°F.

2. Cook butternut squash and water in a saucepan over medium-high heat until soft.

3. Transfer squash and water to a food processor. Add cashews, nutritional yeast, miso, lemon juice, onion powder, salt, and black pepper and blend until smooth. If needed, add more water.

4. Put macaroni in a large baking dish. Pour contents of blender over macaroni and mix well. Season with additional salt. Cover with aluminum foil and bake for 15–20 minutes.

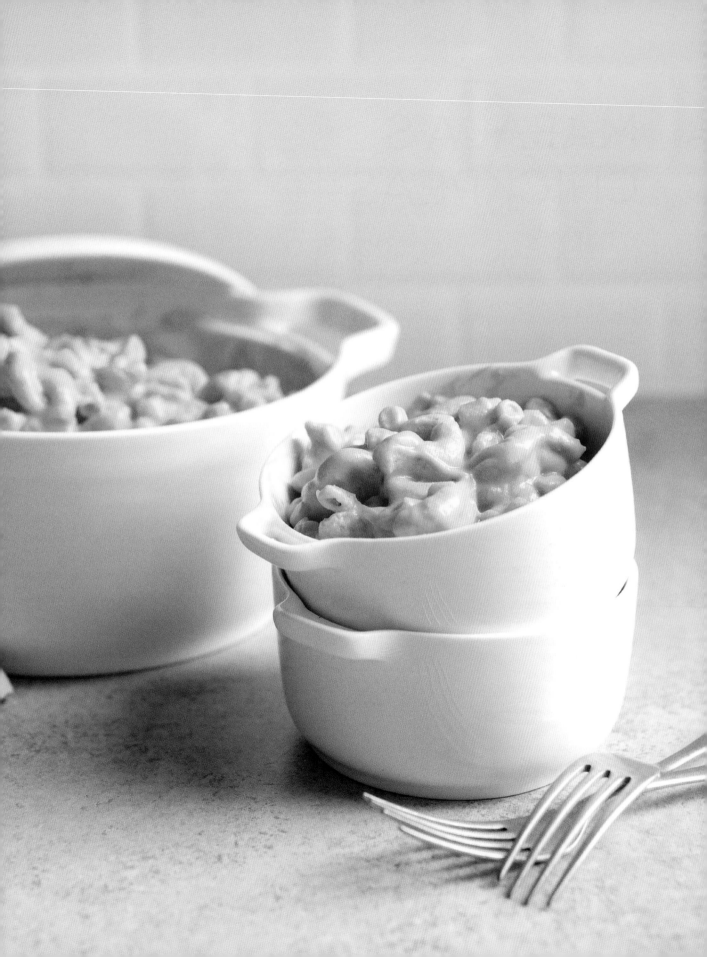

MASALA'S CHICKPEAS

MAKES 6 SERVINGS

This is one of our favorite dishes. We make it often, especially when we travel. If we don't have access to chickpeas, we substitute other vegetables, like spinach, green beans, broccoli, carrots, peppers, snow peas, eggplant, or potatoes. And if we can't locate cumin, coriander, turmeric, and garam masala, we use 3 teaspoons of curry powder.

1 cup diced onions

4 garlic cloves, minced

1 teaspoon grated fresh ginger

2 tablespoons vegetable broth

1 teaspoon ground cumin

1 teaspoon ground coriander

1 teaspoon ground turmeric

½ teaspoon garam masala

2 cups diced tomatoes

2 tablespoons tomato paste

¼ teaspoon cayenne pepper

4 cups cooked or
  canned chickpeas

1 (15-ounce) can lite coconut milk

½ teaspoon lemon juice

Salt, to taste

4 cups cooked brown rice,
  for serving

1. In a large skillet, sauté onions, garlic, and ginger in vegetable broth over medium-high heat until onions brown.

2. Add cumin, coriander, turmeric, and garam masala. Cook for 2–3 minutes.

3. Stir in diced tomatoes, tomato paste, cayenne pepper, chickpeas, and coconut milk.

4. Reduce heat to medium, cover, and cook for 8–10 minutes.

5. Stir in lemon juice and season with salt.

6. Serve on top of rice.

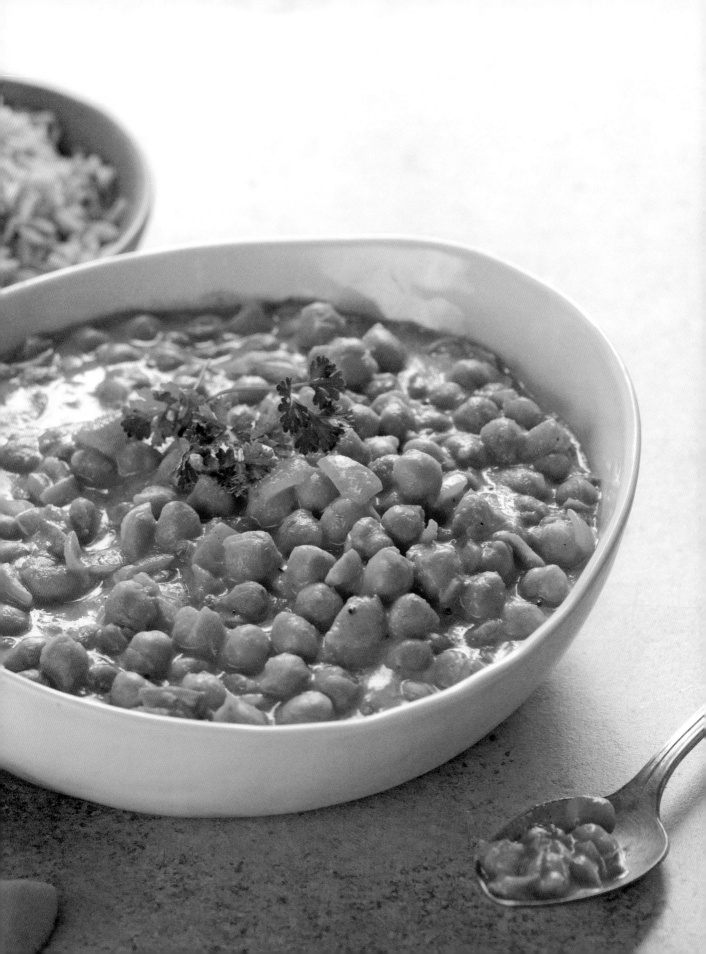

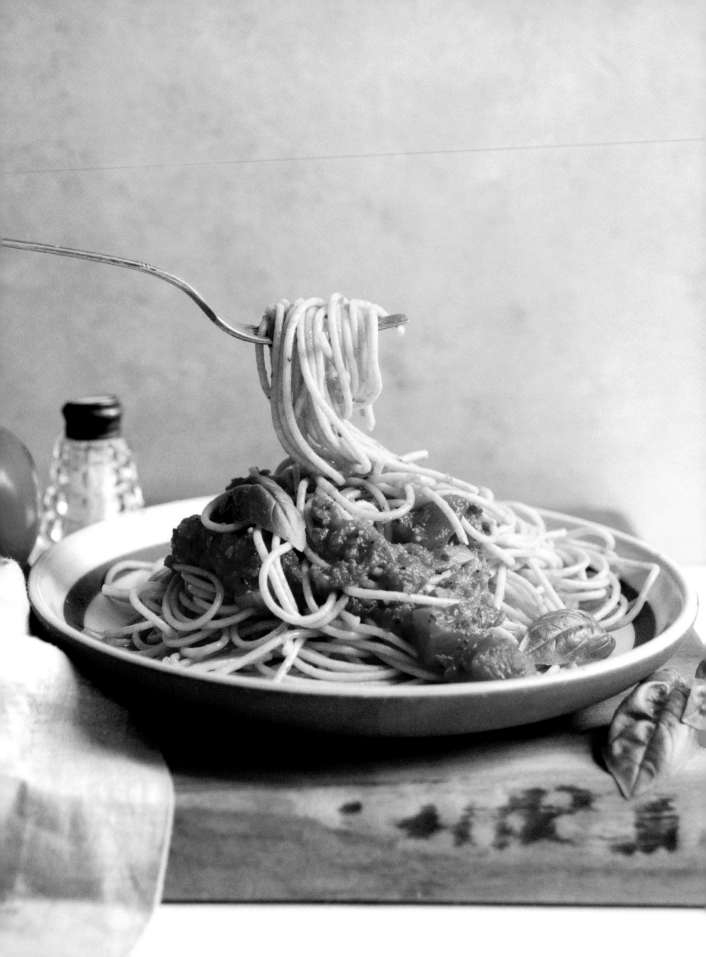

SPAGHETTI WITH FAVORITE MARINARA SAUCE

MAKES 2-3 SERVINGS

This simple sauce takes 5 minutes to prepare and 30–35 minutes to cook on the stovetop. I sometimes like to use my slow cooker for this sauce. I place all the ingredients in the pot, set it on high, and let it cook for 3–4 hours. When using the slow cooker, I double or even triple the recipe.

1 (28-ounce) can diced tomatoes

8 garlic cloves, crushed

1 cup diced onions

1 tablespoon dried oregano

1 tablespoon dried basil

1 teaspoon salt

12 ounces pasta, cooked, for serving

1. In a saucepan, combine tomatoes, garlic, onions, oregano, basil, and salt. Bring to a low simmer, cover, and cook for 30–35 minutes.

2. Transfer to a blender and pulse until mostly smooth but still a bit chunky. Serve over cooked pasta.

NUTTY NOODLES WITH VEGETABLES

MAKES 4 SERVINGS

This tasty dish is simple to prepare. While my spaghetti is cooking, I chop the vegetables, then cook them. I then prepare my sauce, taste it, then balance out the flavors. Snow peas and cauliflower are great additions or replacements for the vegetables called for in this recipe.

—   —

¼ cup vegetable broth

½ onion, sliced

½ red bell pepper, sliced

½ green bell pepper, sliced

½ yellow bell pepper, sliced

2 cups chopped broccoli

1 large carrot, cut into thin strips

½–¾ cup unsweetened nondairy milk (rice, soy, almond, etc.)

½ cup natural peanut butter

⅓ cup reduced-sodium soy sauce

2 tablespoons rice vinegar

1½ teaspoons ground ginger

½ teaspoon raw cane sugar

¼ teaspoon hot sauce

1 pound whole wheat spaghetti or other pasta, cooked

¼ cup crushed peanuts, for garnish

Lime wedges, for garnish

½ cup chopped fresh Thai basil, for garnish

1. In a large skillet, combine vegetable broth, onion, bell peppers, broccoli, and carrot. Cover and cook over medium-high heat for 3–5 minutes, until vegetables are slightly cooked and still crunchy. Do not overcook the vegetables.

2. In a small saucepan, combine ½ cup of milk, peanut butter, soy sauce, rice vinegar, ginger, sugar, and hot sauce. Cook over medium heat, stirring constantly, until mixture is smooth. If sauce is too thick, add up to ¼ cup more milk.

3. Pour half of the peanut sauce over the noodles and gently mix until all noodles are coated.

4. Add remaining sauce to the vegetables and then gently fold the vegetables into the noodles.

5. Garnish with peanuts, lime wedges, and fresh basil.

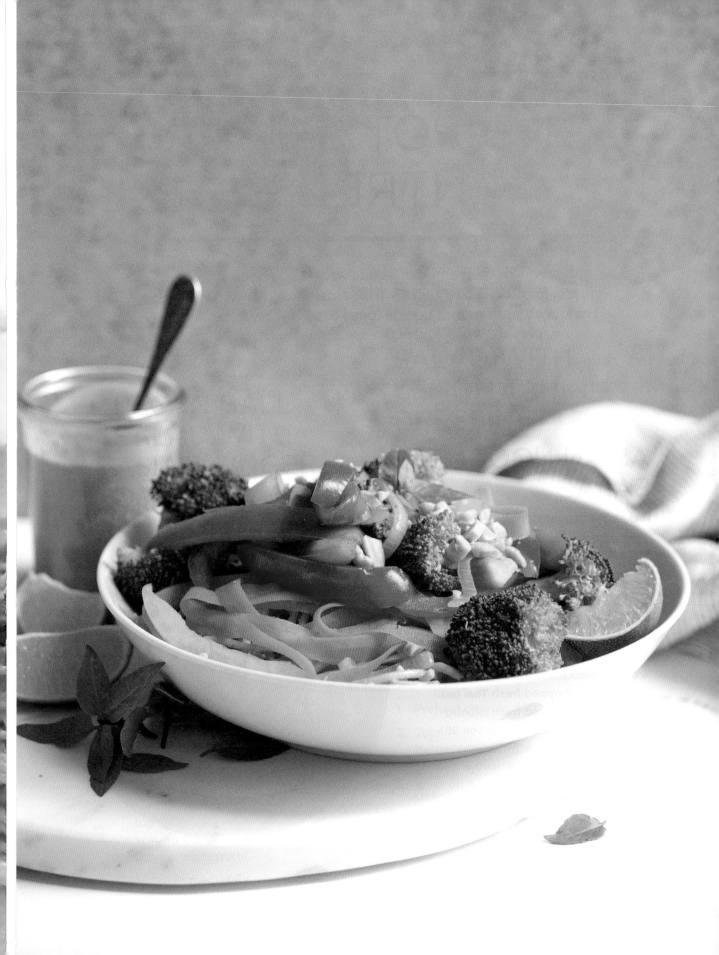

SWEET POTATO ENCHILADAS

MAKES 4–5 SERVINGS

Enchiladas are essentially baked burritos—rolled tortillas filled with savory, tasty fillings, then baked with salsa. I generally use Roasted Tomato Salsa (page 121) with these enchiladas, but you can also use Tomatillo Sauce (page 120).

1 cup diced onions

4 garlic cloves, minced

2 teaspoons ground cumin

1 teaspoon ground coriander

2 tablespoons vegetable broth

2 tablespoons soy sauce

2 cups chopped spinach

2 cups diced cooked
  sweet potatoes

2 cups cooked or canned
  black beans

1 teaspoon salt

10 large tortillas

1 recipe *Roasted Tomato Salsa*
  (page 121) or 1 (16-ounce) jar
  favorite salsa

1. Preheat oven to 350°F.

2. In a large skillet, sauté onions, garlic, cumin, and coriander in vegetable broth over medium-high heat until onions brown.

3. Add soy sauce and spinach. Cover and cook for 2–3 minutes, until spinach wilts. Remove from heat.

4. Fold in sweet potatoes, black beans, and salt.

5. Place ½ cup of mixture in center of each tortilla. Fold in the bottom and sides of each tortilla. Place burritos, seam-side down, in a nonstick baking dish.

6. Pour salsa on top and cover with aluminum foil.

7. Bake for 25 minutes.

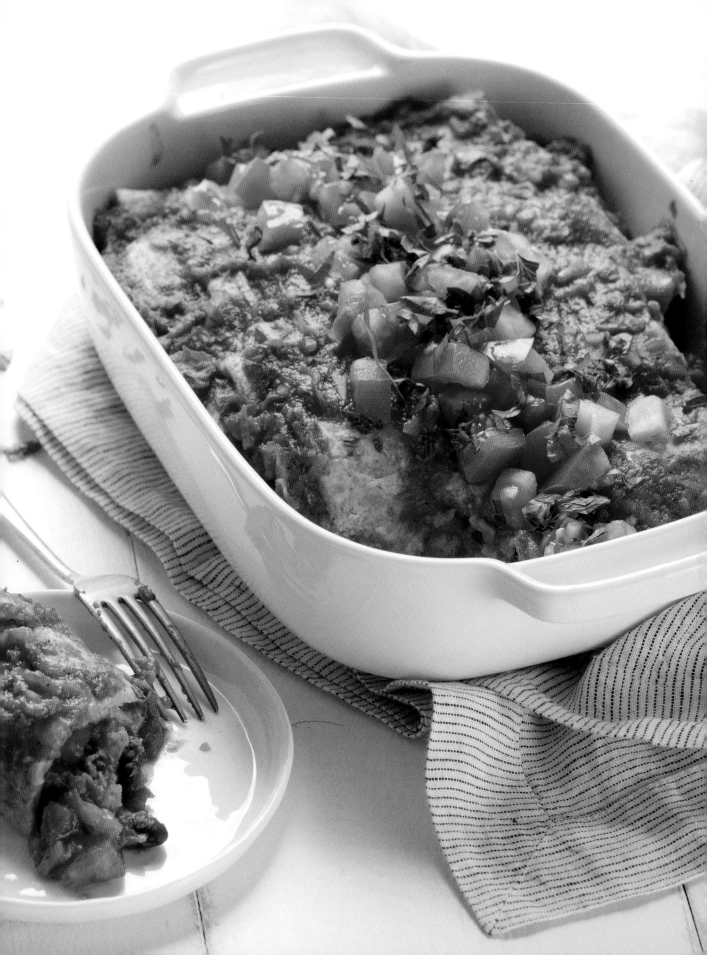

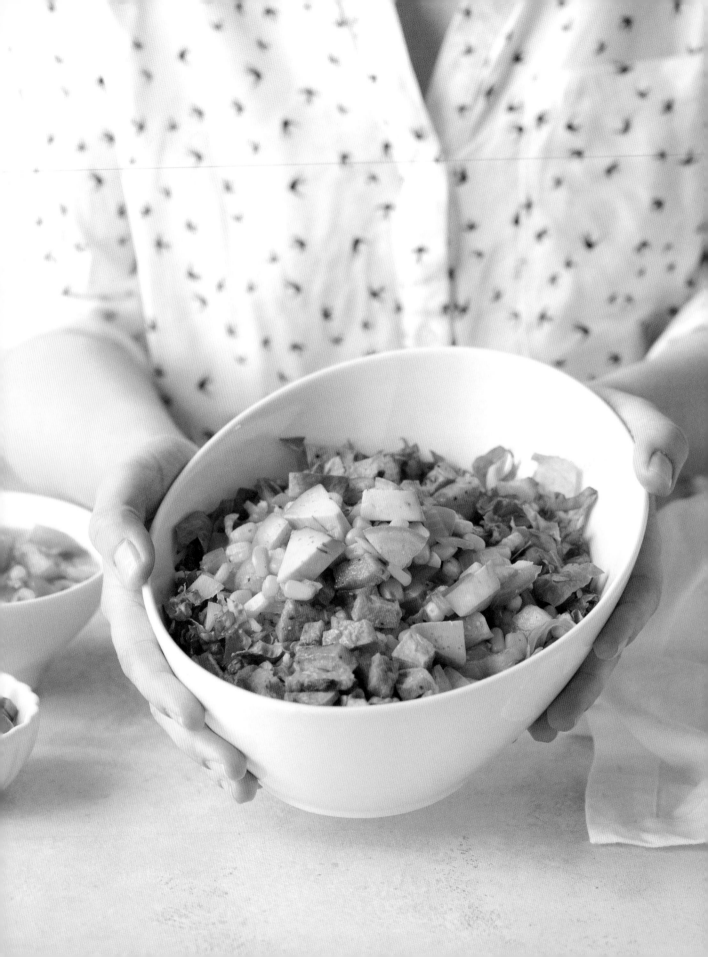

TOMATILLO CORN BOWL

MAKES 4 SERVINGS

This is one of those dishes that you can have two or three times a week and still want more. To satisfy this craving, I often double or triple the sauce recipe, then keep it in my refrigerator or freezer, making it easier and quicker to prepare the next time.

2 large sweet potatoes, diced
Salt and black pepper

Sauce
1 cup onions, diced
4 garlic cloves, minced
2 cups vegetable broth, divided
3 cups corn
2 cups husked, chopped tomatillos
1 jalapeño, seeded and
    coarsely chopped
¼ cup chopped fresh cilantro
1 teaspoon paprika
½ teaspoon onion powder
½ teaspoon dried oregano
½ teaspoon sea salt
2 cups cooked brown rice
4 cups chopped lettuce
Chopped avocados, for garnish

1. Preheat oven to 350°F. Line a baking sheet with parchment.

2. Season sweet potatoes with salt and black pepper and spread on baking sheet. Bake until cooked, about 20 minutes.

3. To prepare sauce, sauté onions and garlic in 2 tablespoons of vegetable broth over medium-high heat until onions brown.

4. Add remaining vegetable broth, corn, tomatillos, and jalapeño. Cook until tomatillos are tender, 5–8 minutes.

5. Add cilantro, paprika, onion powder, oregano, and sea salt. Simmer for 3–5 minutes.

6. Scoop ½ cup of rice in the center of each bowl and circle with chopped lettuce. Add diced potatoes across the bowl and then pour sauce on top. Garnish with avocados.

PUMPKIN GNOCCHI WITH ITALIAN VEGETABLE SAUCE

MAKES 6 SERVINGS

I love taking this dish to pot-lucks. At first, it may seem difficult to make, but it's really quite easy. And once you make it, it becomes easier each time. In fact, you can make almost any type of vegetable gnocchi: potato, sweet potato, beets, etc. I have found tomatoes with jalapeños, zucchinis, and corn to be the perfect topping for pumpkin gnocchi.

1 (15-ounce) can pumpkin puree

2¾ cups whole wheat pastry flour

1 cup sliced onions

1 teaspoon dried basil

1 tablespoon dried oregano

2 tablespoons vegetable broth

1 (28-ounce) can diced tomatoes with jalapeños

2 large zucchinis, sliced

2 cups corn

Salt and black pepper, to taste

1. To make gnocchi, mix pumpkin and flour to make a soft dough. If necessary, add more flour so the dough holds together and is not sticky.

2. Divide dough into 4–5 sections and place on a floured surface. Roll each piece into a rope about 1 inch in diameter. Cut each rope into 1-inch pieces.

3. Fill a large pot with water and salt it generously. Bring to a boil over medium-high heat. Add about one-quarter of the gnocchi to the boiling water and cook until the gnocchi rise to the surface and float, about 5 minutes. With a slotted spoon, remove the gnocchi from the water and transfer to a serving dish. Continue until all the gnocchi are cooked.

4. In a large saucepan, sauté onions, basil, and oregano in vegetable broth over medium-high heat until onions brown. Add tomatoes, zucchinis, and corn. Cover and cook for 5–7 minutes, until zucchini is tender.

5. Place vegetable sauce on top of gnocchi and season with salt and black pepper. Serve immediately.

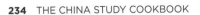

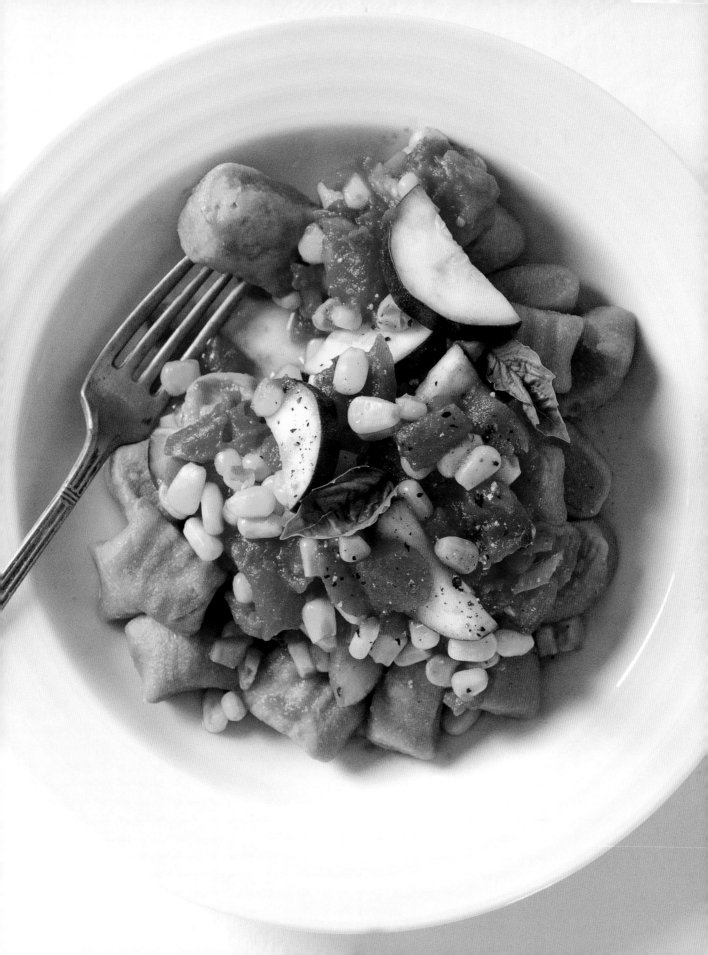

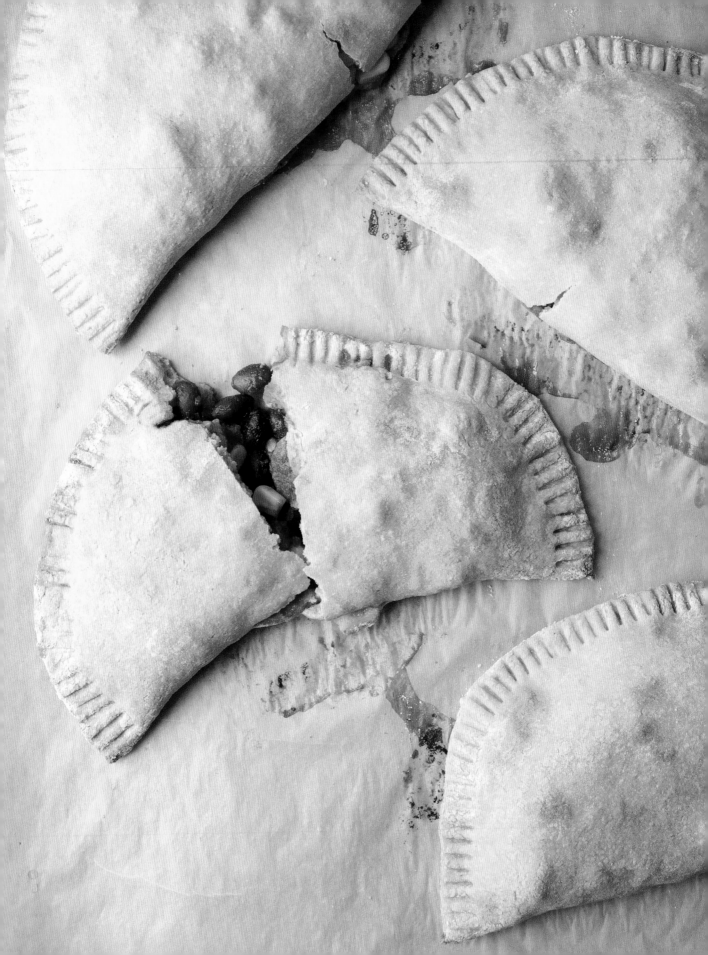

SOUTHWESTERN CALZONES

MAKES 8 CALZONES

I had my first salsa pizza in Rochester, New York, 20 years ago, and I loved it. This is a spin-off of that recipe. Instead of making a pizza shell, we are making calzones and stuffing them with salsa, black beans, corn, onions, and spicy seitan (optional).

Dough
1½ cups warm water

3 teaspoons instant yeast

1 tablespoon maple syrup

4 cups whole wheat pastry flour

½ teaspoon salt

Filling
1 (15-ounce) jar salsa

2 cups corn

1 can cooked or canned
    black beans

¼ cup diced onions

1 (4-ounce) package spicy
    seitan, cut into bite-size pieces
    (optional)

1. For the dough, whisk together warm water, yeast, and maple syrup in a large bowl. Let set for 5 minutes, until the mixture begins to foam. Add the flour and salt. Knead with your hands for 5–6 minutes, until smooth and elastic.

2. Cut the dough into eight equal pieces. Roll the dough into smooth balls and place in a nonstick baking pan about 2 inches apart. Cover with plastic wrap and set in a warm, draft-free area for 1 hour.

3. Preheat oven to 425°F. Line a baking sheet with parchment.

4. In a large bowl, mix all filling ingredients.

5. On a lightly floured surface, roll each dough ball into a circle about 6 inches in diameter. Place 2–3 heaping tablespoons of filling in the center of the circle. Wet the edges of the dough with a little water and pinch the sides together.

6. Place calzones on lined baking sheet and bake for 20–30 minutes, until tops are lightly browned.

7. Serve hot.

STUFFED EGGPLANT
WITH SUN-DRIED TOMATO SAUCE

MAKES 6 SERVINGS

When people in the Dominican Republic make stuffed eggplant, they remove the top stem, then cut out the insides of the eggplant. I find this a bit hard, so I cut them in half lengthwise. I have filled them with potatoes and cauliflower, but my favorite is spinach macaroni, topped with sun-dried tomato sauce.

4 eggplants
Salt, for rubbing

Spinach Macaroni Filling
½ cup chopped onions
4 garlic cloves, minced
2 tablespoons vegetable broth
½ teaspoon dried oregano
½ teaspoon dried basil
¾ cup water
2 cups finely chopped cooked spinach
½ teaspoon salt
1½ cups cooked macaroni

Tomato Water
¾ cup water
2 tablespoons tomato paste
½ tablespoon lemon juice
¼ teaspoon salt

Sun-Dried Tomato Sauce
¼ cup chopped onions
4 garlic cloves, minced
3½ cups finely diced tomatoes
¼ cup minced sun-dried tomatoes (without oil)
2 teaspoons dried oregano
2 teaspoons dried basil
1 teaspoon salt
1 teaspoon cane sugar

1. Preheat oven to 350°F.

2. Cut eggplants in half lengthwise, then scoop out the flesh, leaving a ½-inch-thick shell along the sides. Dice the scooped-out flesh and reserve 1 cup for the filling.

3. Lightly rub salt on the insides of the eggplants. Place eggplants in a casserole dish and set aside.

4. In a large skillet, sauté onions and garlic in vegetable broth over medium-high heat, until onions brown.

5. Add oregano, basil, water, spinach, diced eggplant, and salt. Sauté until eggplant is tender. Fold in cooked macaroni.

6. Spoon 3–4 heaping tablespoons of spinach macaroni filling into each eggplant half.

7. Prepare tomato water by whisking together water, tomato paste, lemon juice, and salt. Pour into casserole dish around eggplant.

8. Bake, uncovered, for 25–30 minutes.

9. While eggplants are baking, prepare sun-dried tomato sauce.

10. Dry sauté onions and garlic over medium-high heat in nonstick skillet.

11. Add diced tomatoes, sun-dried tomatoes, oregano, basil, salt, and sugar. Cover and cook for 20 minutes, until tomatoes cook down.

12. Serve tomato sauce on top of stuffed eggplants.

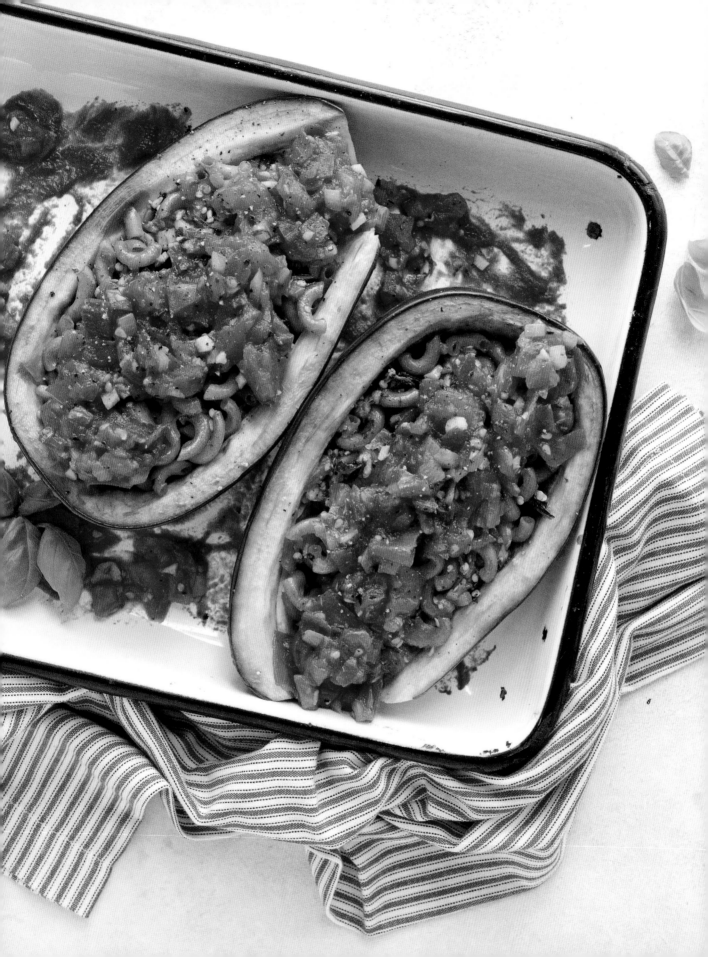

THAI VEGETABLE CURRY

MAKES 4 SERVINGS

This simple, tasty dish can be prepared with a wide range of vegetables. I often make it at the end of the week, using whatever vegetables remain in my refrigerator. It's slightly different each time, but always tasty.

1 cup sliced onions

4 garlic cloves, minced

2 teaspoons grated fresh ginger

2 tablespoons minced jalapeño

2 tablespoons vegetable broth

2 cups lite canned coconut milk

2 tablespoons reduced-sodium
soy sauce

1½ teaspoons Thai red curry paste

1 teaspoon lime juice

2 cups chopped broccoli, steamed

1 cup green beans, steamed

½ red bell pepper, sliced, steamed

2 cups chopped spinach, steamed

1 cup fresh basil, loosely packed

Cooked brown rice, for serving

Peanuts, for garnish

Lime wedges, for garnish

1. In a large pot, sauté onions, garlic, ginger, and jalapeño in vegetable broth over medium-high heat for 3–4 minutes, until onions are browned.

2. Add coconut milk, soy sauce, curry paste, and lime juice. Bring to a low simmer.

3. Fold in steamed vegetables and basil. Cook for 1 minute. I generally like my vegetables crunchy, but if you want, cook 1–5 minutes longer.

4. Serve over brown rice, garnished with peanuts and lime wedges.

note: If I don't have Thai red curry paste on hand, I replace it with 1 teaspoon ground cumin, 1 teaspoon ground coriander, 1 teaspoon ground turmeric, and ½ teaspoon of garam masala.

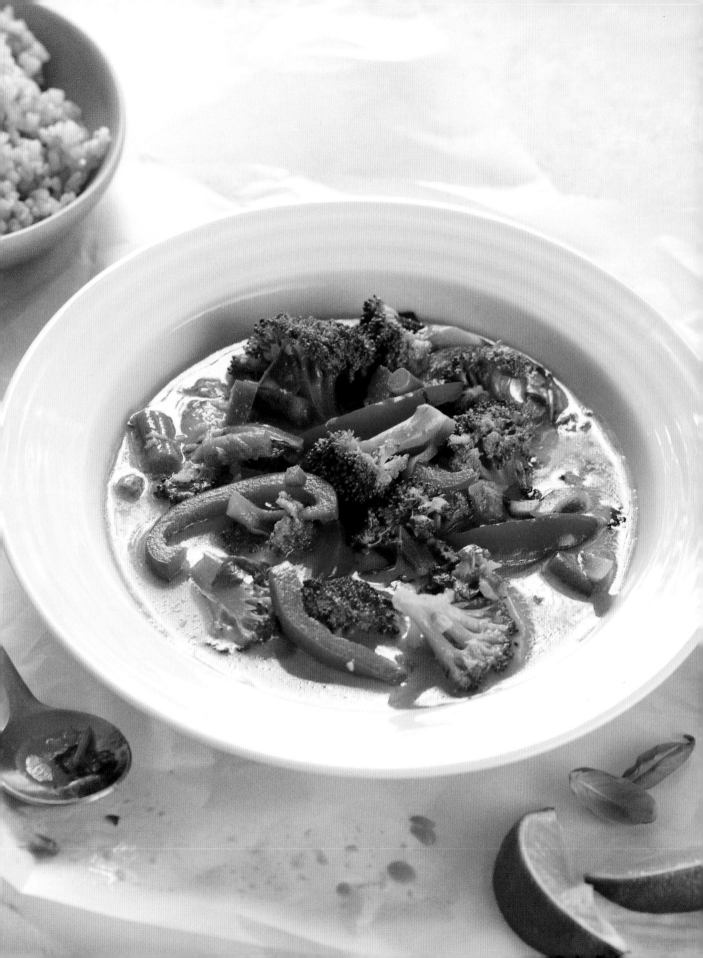

TOMATILLO TORTILLA BAKE

MAKES 6 SERVINGS

It's fine to use store-bought baked tortilla chips for this recipe, but I often make my own. I place 8 lightly salted corn tortillas on a baking sheet and bake at 350° for 5–8 minutes. Since they are easy to burn, I check them often. Once they are hard and crunchy, I let them cool for 10 minutes before crumbling them.

 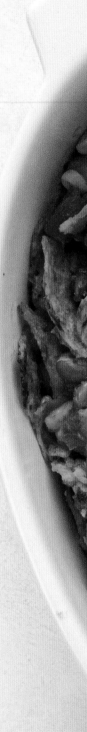

3 cups crumbled baked corn tortilla chips

2 (15-ounce) jars salsa

2 cups corn

2 cups cooked or canned pinto beans

1½ cups *Tomatillo Sauce* **(page 120)**

Diced avocados, for garnish

1. Preheat oven to 350°F.

2. In a mixing bowl, combine crumbled tortilla chips, salsa, corn, and beans. Mix well. Spread in the bottom of a 9 × 13-inch nonstick baking dish. Cover with aluminum foil and bake for 30 minutes.

3. Remove the tortilla bake from the oven and let cool for 15 minutes. Drizzle with tomatillo sauce and top with avocado.

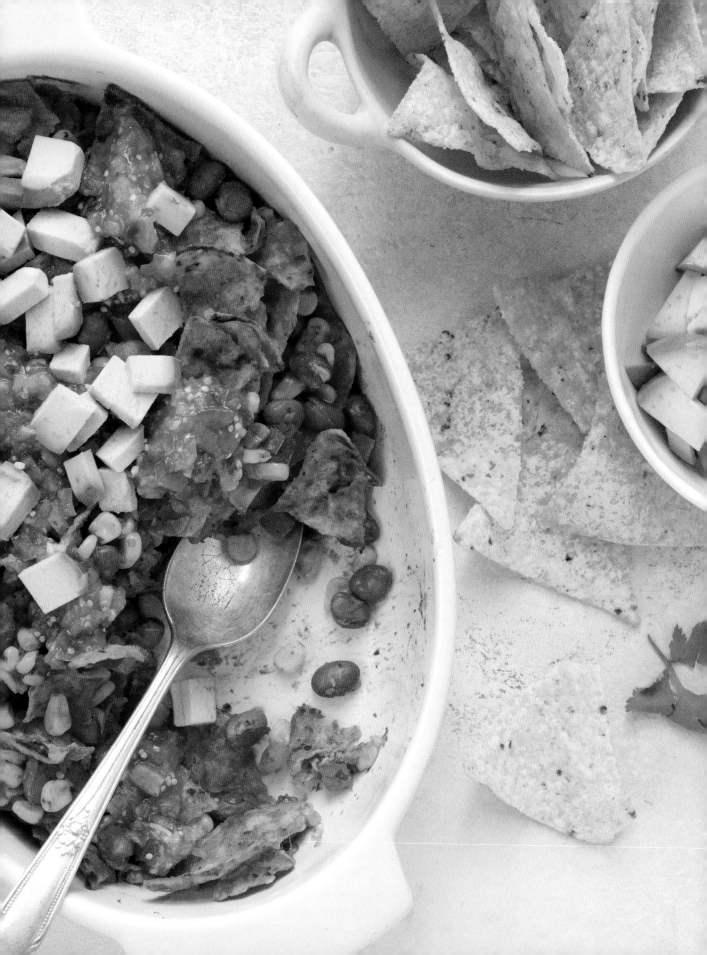

VEGETABLE DUMPLING STEW

MAKES 6 SERVINGS

Chicken with dumplings was one of my favorite childhood dishes. My mother would fill our bowls with long homemade noodles made with eggs and white flour. In this recipe, I've made my own version of this childhood dish. I've used mixed vegetables in place of chicken and nondairy milk and whole wheat flour in place of eggs and white flour.

Stew

1 cup diced onions

4 garlic cloves, minced

4 cups vegetable broth, divided

½ teaspoon dried oregano

½ teaspoon dried basil

½ teaspoon dried thyme

1 cup diced potatoes

¼ cup chopped fresh parsley

½ cup peas

½ cup corn

½ cup chopped green beans

½ cup chopped carrots

Salt and black pepper, to taste

Dumplings

1½ cups whole wheat pastry flour

½ teaspoon baking soda

Pinch of salt

1 teaspoon raw cane sugar

¾ cup unsweetened nondairy milk (rice, soy, almond, etc.)

1. For the stew, in a large saucepan, sauté onions and garlic in 2 tablespoons of vegetable broth over medium-high heat until onions brown.

2. Add remaining vegetable broth, oregano, basil, thyme, and potatoes. Bring to a simmer, cover, and cook until potatoes are tender.

3. Add parsley, peas, corn, green beans, and carrots. Reduce heat, cover, and cook for an additional 10 minutes, until vegetables are tender. Season with salt and black pepper.

4. For the dumplings, mix flour, baking soda, salt, and sugar. Add milk and stir until dry mixture is moistened.

5. Gently drop dough by rounded tablespoons into simmering stew. Cook, uncovered, over low heat for 10 minutes. Then cover and cook for 7–10 more minutes, until dumplings are cooked through.

6. Serve immediately.

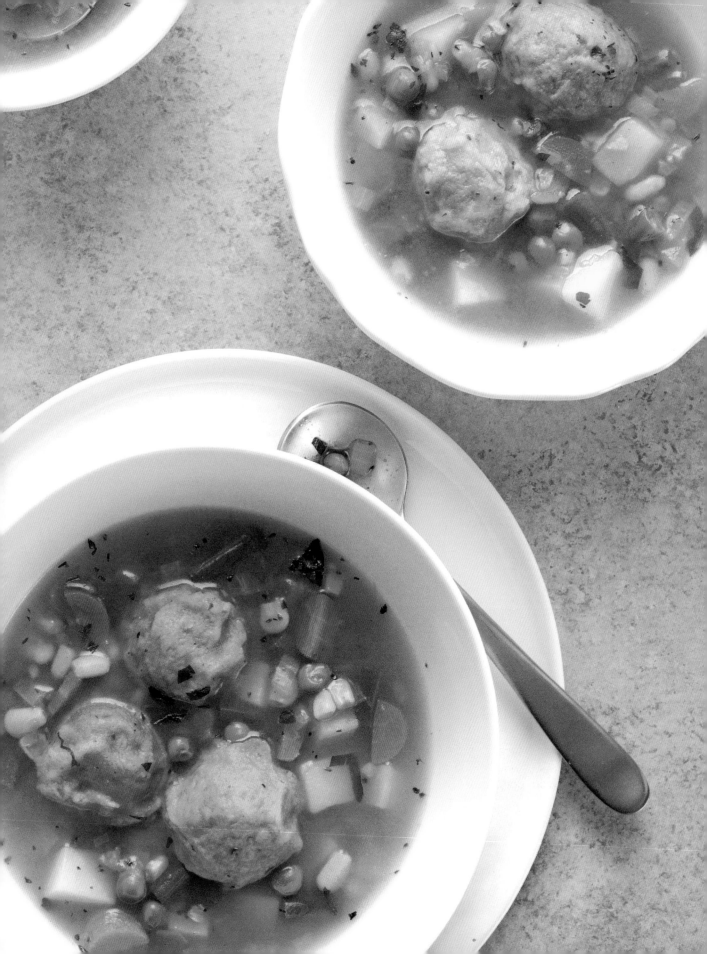

VEGETABLE LASAGNA

MAKES 6 SERVINGS

This lasagna has always been one of our go-to meals. I would make a large pan of it, with the intention of having leftovers for school lunches the next day. But if I didn't take out the school lunch servings before sitting down, my sons would eat the entire pan, going back three or even four times!

1 (14-ounce) package extra-firm tofu, crumbled
5 cups spinach
4 garlic cloves, minced
1 tablespoon dried oregano
1 tablespoon dried basil
½ teaspoon salt
8 cups *Favorite Marinara Sauce* (page 221)
1 pound lasagna noodles

1. Preheat oven to 350°F.

2. Combine tofu, spinach, garlic, oregano, basil, and salt in a large bowl. Mix well.

3. Spread ½ cup of marinara sauce over the bottom of a 9 × 13-inch baking dish. Layer with one-third of the uncooked noodles, then top with half of the tofu mixture and ½–1 cup of marinara sauce. Top with another layer of noodles, remaining tofu mixture, and another layer of marinara sauce. Finish with a third layer of noodles and the remaining sauce.

4. Cover with aluminum foil and bake for 1 hour. Wait 10 minutes before serving.

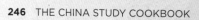

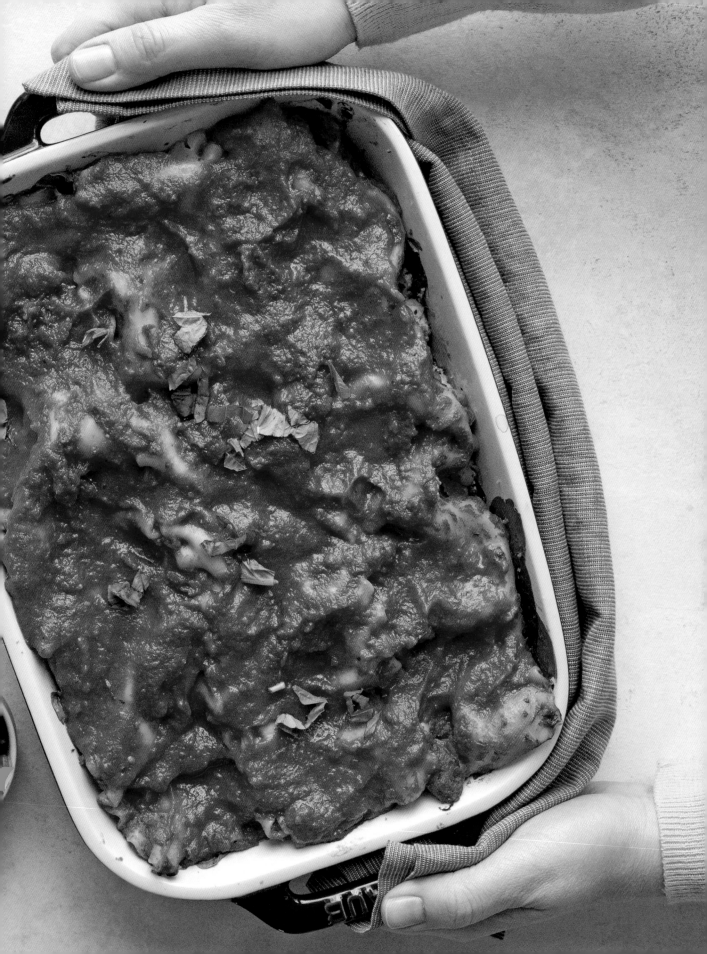

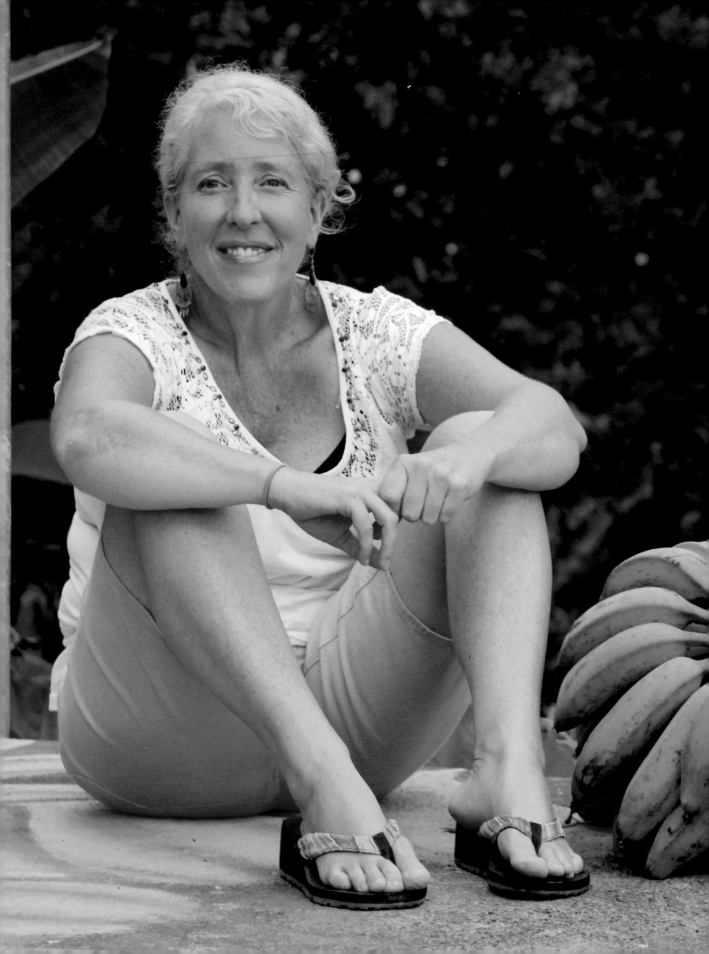

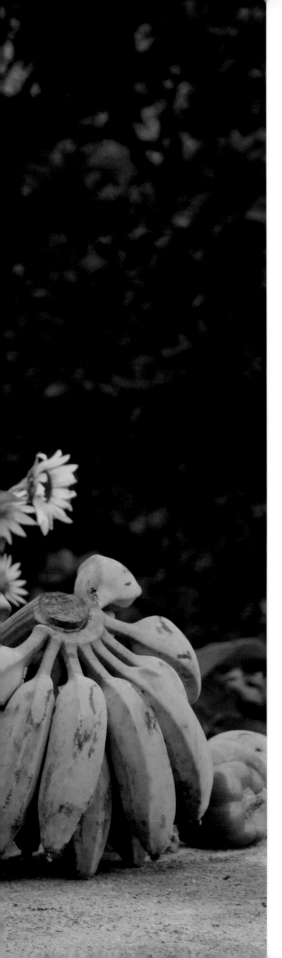

SIDES

BAKED BEANS

MAKES 3-4 SERVINGS

When I was younger, I was not a big fan of baked beans. But my mother was, and she made them often. It wasn't until I visited England and had my first baked potato topped with baked beans, and beans on toast, that I became a fan as well. I usually double this recipe since these beans are good as leftovers.

¼ cup diced onions

1 (15-ounce) can navy beans, rinsed and drained

½ cup tomato sauce

2 tablespoons maple syrup

1 teaspoon apple cider vinegar

1 teaspoon Dijon mustard

2 tablespoons diced dill pickles

¼ teaspoon salt

1. Preheat oven to 350°F.

2. Place onions, beans, tomato sauce, maple syrup, vinegar, mustard, dill pickles, and salt in a casserole dish and mix well.

3. Cover and bake for 25–30 minutes.

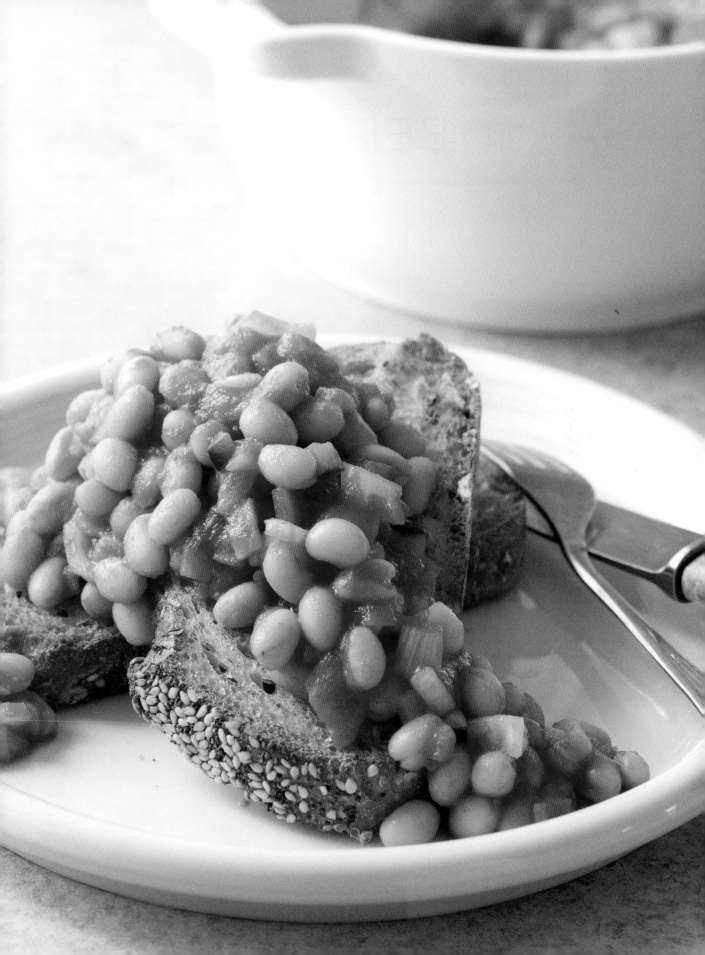

BEETS

We love beets, and like most vegetables, they can be cooked in many different ways. The first recipe is a mustard-flavored dish that goes well with Caribbean Moro (page 256). The second is a more traditional pickled beet dish that goes well with salads.

MUSTAFA'S BEETS WITH MUSTARD AND DILL

MAKES 3–4 SERVINGS

4 medium beets
1 tablespoon lemon juice
1 tablespoon reduced-sodium soy sauce
1½ teaspoons Dijon mustard
¼ teaspoon dried dill or 1½ teaspoons chopped fresh dill

1. Wash beets and cut off the tops.

2. Bring a pot of water to a boil over medium-high heat. Add beets and cook for 30 minutes, until tender. Drain.

3. When the beets are cool enough to handle, peel them and slice into ¼-inch-thick rounds. Transfer beets to a saucepan.

4. In a small bowl, whisk together lemon juice, soy sauce, mustard, and dill. Pour over beets and cook for 2 minutes.

5. Serve warm.

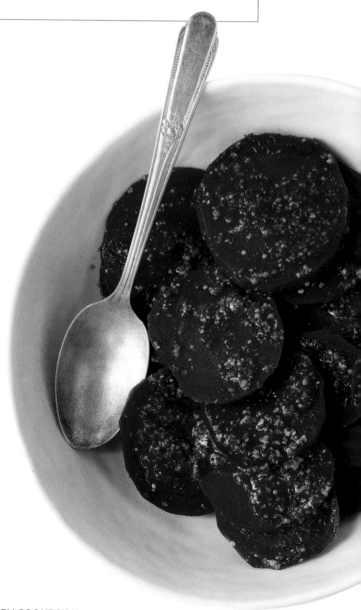

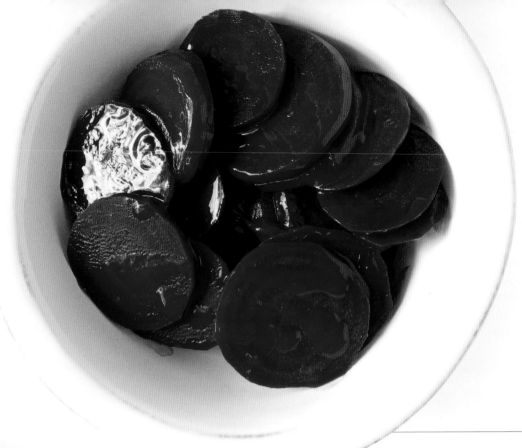

HARVARD BEETS

MAKES 3-4 SERVINGS

4 medium beets
2 tablespoons apple cider vinegar
1 tablespoon maple syrup
1½ teaspoons cornstarch
Salt, to taste

1. Wash beets and cut off the tops.

2. Bring a pot of water to a boil over medium-high heat. Add beets and cook for 30 minutes, until tender. Drain.

3. When the beets are cool enough to handle, peel them and slice into ¼-inch-thick rounds. Transfer beets to a saucepan.

4. In a small bowl, whisk together vinegar, maple syrup, cornstarch, and salt. Pour over beets and cook for 2 minutes.

5. Serve warm.

CAULIFLOWER

I often serve one of these cauliflower dishes with one or two other side dishes. The first recipe is a good replacement for mashed potatoes. The second is a simple sauté, and the last has a tangy tomato flavor. The first two dishes go well with Garlic Green Beans with Mushrooms (page 265) and "Oyster" Flavored Bok Choy (page 269). The last goes well with *Plátanos Maduros* (page 267) and Caribbean Moro (page 256).

CREAMED CAULIFLOWER

MAKES 3-4 SERVINGS

4 cups chopped cauliflower
½ cup vegetable broth
½ cup raw cashews
2 tablespoons nutritional yeast
1 tablespoon white miso
Sea salt and black pepper, to taste

1. Preheat oven to 350°F.

2. Place cauliflower in a medium saucepan and pour in an inch of water. Cover and cook over medium-high heat until soft. Drain and transfer to a 9 × 9-inch baking dish.

3. Place vegetable broth, cashews, nutritional yeast, and white miso in a food processor. Process until smooth and creamy.

4. Mix sauce with cauliflower. Season with salt and black pepper.

5. Bake, uncovered, for 7–10 minutes.

6. Serve warm.

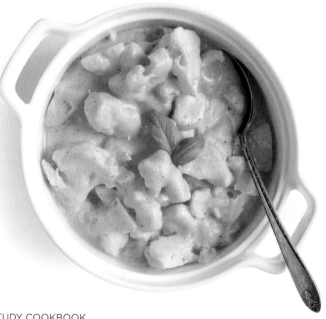

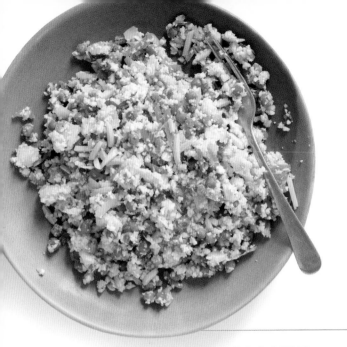

CURRIED CAULIFLOWER WITH TOMATOES

MAKES 3-4 SERVINGS

3 garlic cloves, minced

1 teaspoon ground coriander

1 teaspoon ground cumin

4 cups chopped cauliflower

2 cups diced tomatoes

1 cup water

1 tablespoon tomato paste

1 tablespoon lemon juice

1 teaspoon salt

Cayenne pepper, to taste

In a large skillet, dry sauté garlic, coriander, and cumin over medium-high heat for 1–2 minutes. Add cauliflower, tomatoes, water, tomato paste, lemon juice, salt, and cayenne pepper. Cover and cook for 6–7 minutes, until cauliflower is soft but not mushy.

CAULIFLOWER SAUTÉ

MAKES 3-4 SERVINGS

½ cup diced onions

4 garlic cloves, minced

4 tablespoons vegetable broth, divided

⅓ cup grated carrots

6 cups cauliflower florets, pulsed in a food processor into rice-size pieces

1 cup frozen peas

1 teaspoon salt

¼ cup slivered almonds

2 tablespoons minced fresh basil

4 teaspoons lemon juice

1. In a large skillet, sauté onions and garlic in 1 tablespoon of vegetable broth over medium-high heat until onions brown.

2. Add remaining vegetable broth, carrots, cauliflower, peas, and salt. Cover and cook over medium-low heat for 3–5 minutes, until softened. Remove from heat.

3. Stir in almonds and basil. Sprinkle with lemon juice.

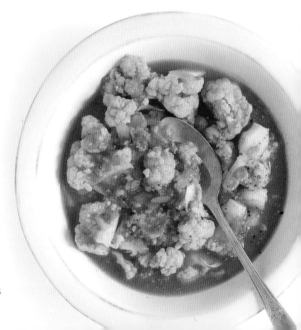

CARIBBEAN MORO

MAKES 4 SERVINGS

This is one of the first dishes my sons learned to cook. It's a great base dish, meaning that the beans can be replaced with equal amounts of other vegetables, such as corn, green beans, diced carrots, or peas. And what's more, leftovers make great burrito fillings, together with grilled vegetables, salsa, and Golden Cheese Sauce (page 171).

1 medium onion, diced

3 garlic cloves, minced

½ green bell pepper, diced

¼ cup chopped fresh cilantro

2 tablespoons vegetable broth

2½ cups water

1 cup brown rice

1 (15-ounce) can pigeon peas, pinto beans, or black beans, rinsed and drained

1 rounded tablespoon tomato paste

½ teaspoon salt, plus more to taste

1. In a medium-size saucepan, sauté onion, garlic, green pepper, and cilantro in vegetable broth over medium-high heat until onion and peppers brown.

2. Add water, rice, beans, tomato paste, and salt.

3. Bring to a boil, then reduce heat to low and cover. Cook for 30–40 minutes, until water is absorbed and rice is tender. Season with salt.

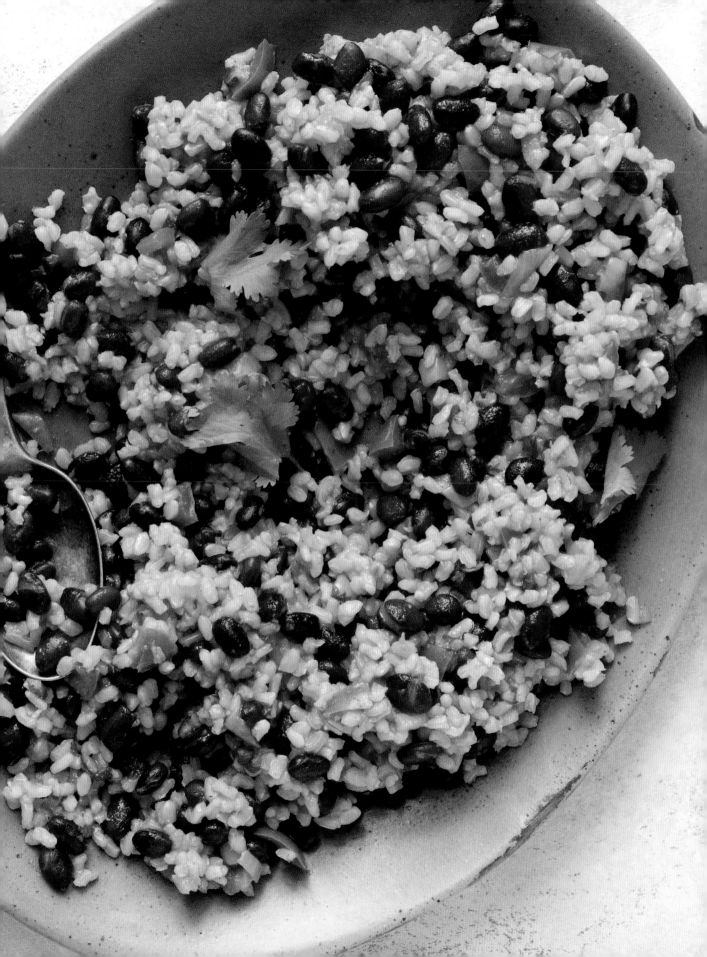

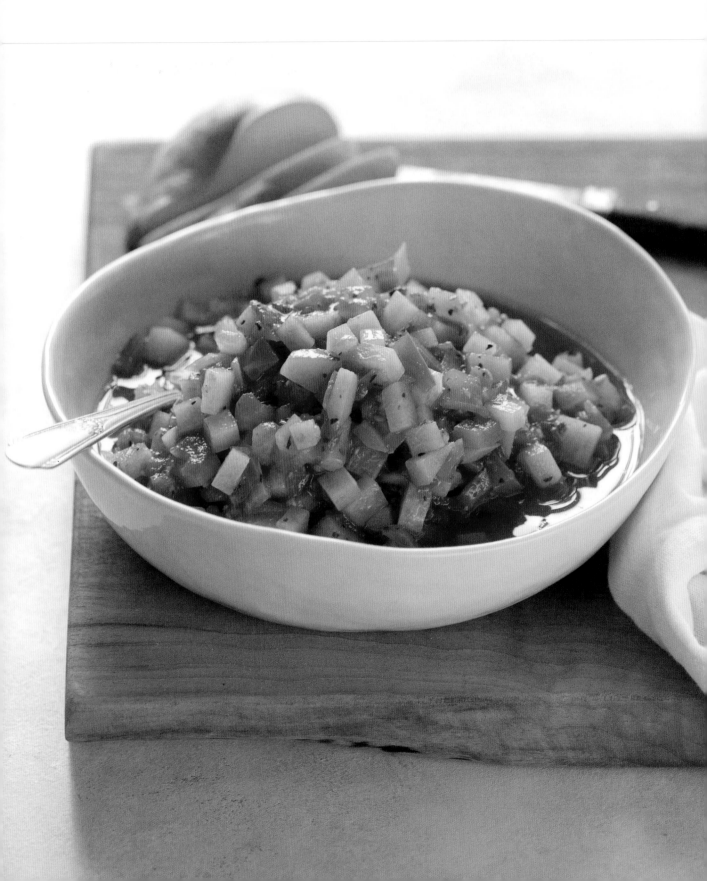

CHAYOTE GUISADO

MAKES 4 SERVINGS

Growing on a treetop vine, chayotes are pear-shaped light green squashes that can be eaten raw or cooked in many different ways—boiled, fried, sautéed, etc. Chayotes have a relatively mellow taste, taking on the flavors of the seasonings in which they are cooked, and can be found in most grocery stores.

2 medium chayotes

¼ cup diced onions

3 garlic cloves, minced

¼ cup diced green bell peppers

2 tablespoons vegetable broth

1 cup water

2 cups finely diced tomatoes

2 tablespoons tomato paste

1 tablespoon dried oregano

1 tablespoon lemon juice

Salt and black pepper, to taste

1. Peel each chayote, slice it down the middle, remove the inner core, and dice it into small pieces. You should have about 4 cups. Set aside.

2. In a large skillet, sauté onions, garlic, and bell peppers in vegetable broth over medium-high heat until onions brown.

3. Add water, chayotes, tomatoes, tomato paste, oregano, and lemon juice. Cover and cook for 15–20 minutes, until chayotes are soft. If necessary, add additional water. Season with salt and black pepper.

CORN

During our teacher study tours to Guanajuato, Mexico, we had a favorite street vendor who sold corn on the cob. With lots of toppings to choose from, we were able to create a wide range of flavorful cobs. Several of these flavors are replicated in these recipes using chili powder, lime, basil, cayenne pepper, and nutritional yeast in place of grated cotija cheese.

BASIL PEPPER CORN

MAKES 3–4 SERVINGS

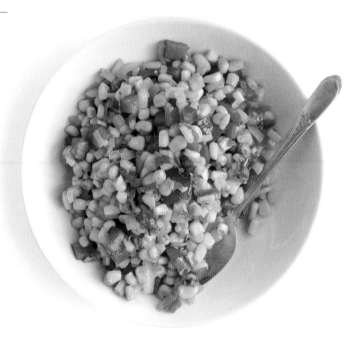

1 medium onion, diced

2 garlic cloves, minced

2 tablespoons vegetable broth

1 red bell pepper, seeded and diced

2½ cups corn, fresh off the cob

1 rounded tablespoon chopped fresh basil

Salt and cayenne pepper, to taste

In a large skillet, sauté onion and garlic in vegetable broth over medium-high heat until onion browns. Add bell pepper, corn, and basil. Cook for 3–4 minutes. Season with salt and cayenne pepper.

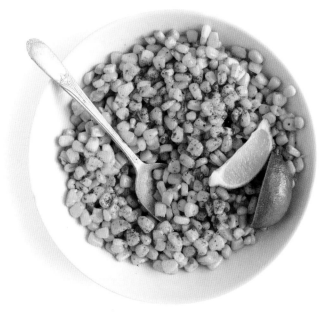

CHILI LIME CORN

MAKES 3-4 SERVINGS

2½ cups corn, fresh off the cob
½ teaspoon chili powder
2 teaspoons lime juice
2 tablespoons vegetable broth
1 tablespoon nutritional yeast
Salt, to taste

In a large skillet, sauté corn, chili powder, and lime juice in vegetable broth over medium-high heat for 3–5 minutes. Add nutritional yeast and season with salt.

COCONUT CREAMED CORN

MAKES 3-4 SERVINGS

½ medium onion, diced
2 tablespoons vegetable broth
2½ cups corn, fresh off the cob
1 cup lite coconut milk mixed with
   2 teaspoons cornstarch
2 tablespoons nutritional yeast
Salt and black pepper, to taste

In a large skillet, sauté onion in vegetable broth over medium-high heat until brown. Add corn, milk with cornstarch, and nutritional yeast. Cook for 3–5 minutes. Season with salt and black pepper.

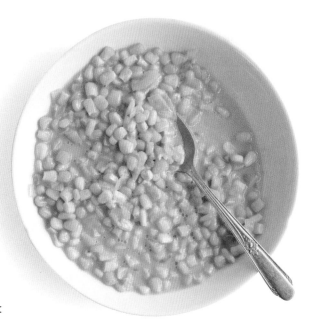

CRANBERRY APPLESAUCE

MAKES 3-4 SERVINGS

Living in Upstate New York, we always had lots of apples, and it was fun to find new ways to prepare applesauce. We used it as an oil/butter replacement in cakes, muffins, and quick breads and served it on our pancakes at breakfast.

1 cup fresh cranberries
3 cups peeled, chopped apples
½ cup unsweetened apple juice concentrate
½ cup water
1 teaspoon ground cinnamon
2 tablespoons maple syrup

1. Combine cranberries, apples, apple juice concentrate, water, and cinnamon in a saucepan. Cover and cook over medium heat until cranberries and apples are soft. The cooking time will vary depending on the type of apple used, taking anywhere from 8–20 minutes.

2. Drain off liquid, then transfer to a food processor. Pulse 5–6 times.

3. Transfer to a serving bowl.

4. Add maple syrup and serve warm.

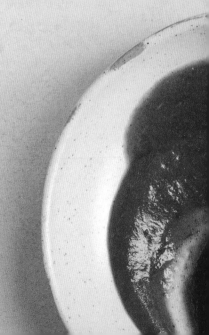

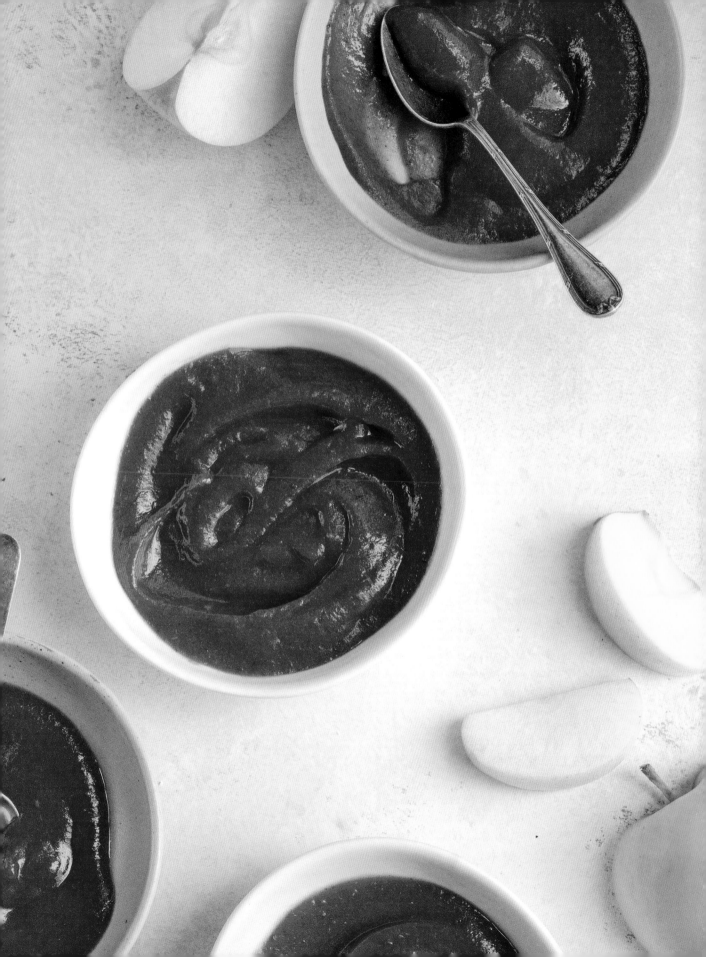

GREEN BEANS

Green beans are popular in our house, so I plant them each spring in our garden. Occasionally, we're out of town when they are ready to be picked, and we come home to find large overgrown beans. Yes, they are big and tough, but with the Cilantro Green Beans recipe, I'm still able to enjoy them. However, with the Garlic Green Beans and the Fasolia recipes, I prefer to use tender fresh beans. I like to serve Fasolia on baked potatoes and Garlic Green Beans with pasta.

CILANTRO GREEN BEANS

MAKES 3-4 SERVINGS

1 large onion, diced
2 teaspoons minced garlic
½ green bell pepper, diced
¼ cup chopped fresh cilantro
¼ cup vegetable broth, divided
3 cups finely diced green beans
Salt and black pepper, to taste

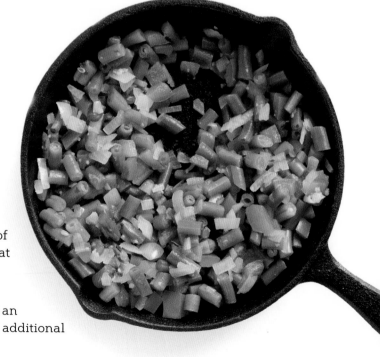

1. In a skillet, sauté onion, garlic, bell pepper, and cilantro in 2 tablespoons of vegetable broth over medium-high heat until onion browns.

2. Add remaining vegetable broth and diced green beans. Cover and cook for an additional 3–5 minutes. If needed, add additional vegetable broth.

3. Season with salt and black pepper. Serve warm.

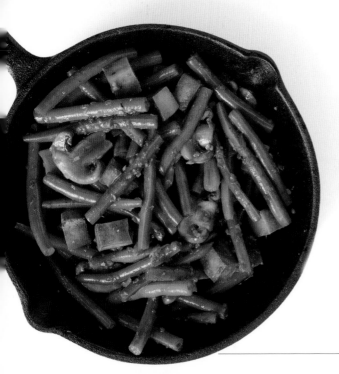

FASOLIA (ETHIOPIAN GREEN BEANS AND CARROTS)

MAKES 3–4 SERVINGS

1 medium onion, chopped

3 garlic cloves, minced

1 teaspoon grated fresh ginger

½ teaspoon ground turmeric

2 tablespoons vegetable broth

4 cups pureed tomatoes

3 cups chopped green beans

1 cup chopped carrots

Salt, to taste

1. Sauté onion, garlic, ginger, and turmeric in vegetable broth over medium-high heat until onion browns.

2. Add tomatoes, green beans, and carrots. Cover and cook for 4–5 minutes. Season with salt.

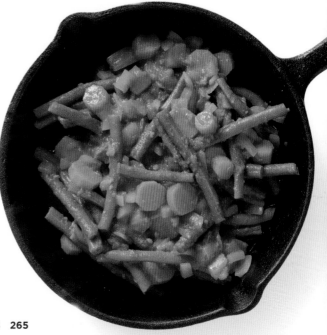

GARLIC GREEN BEANS WITH MUSHROOMS

MAKES 3-4 SERVINGS

¼ cup vegetable broth

6 garlic cloves, minced

3 cups green beans

2 cups sliced mushrooms (portobello or button)

2 tablespoons reduced-sodium soy sauce mixed with 1 teaspoon cornstarch

Salt and black pepper, to taste

½ cup cubed *Baked Tofu* (page 95)

1. In a skillet, combine vegetable broth, garlic, and green beans. Cover and cook over medium-high heat for 2–3 minutes.

2. Add mushrooms and soy sauce with cornstarch. Cover and cook for 3–4 minutes.

3. Season with salt and pepper, then add tofu and serve.

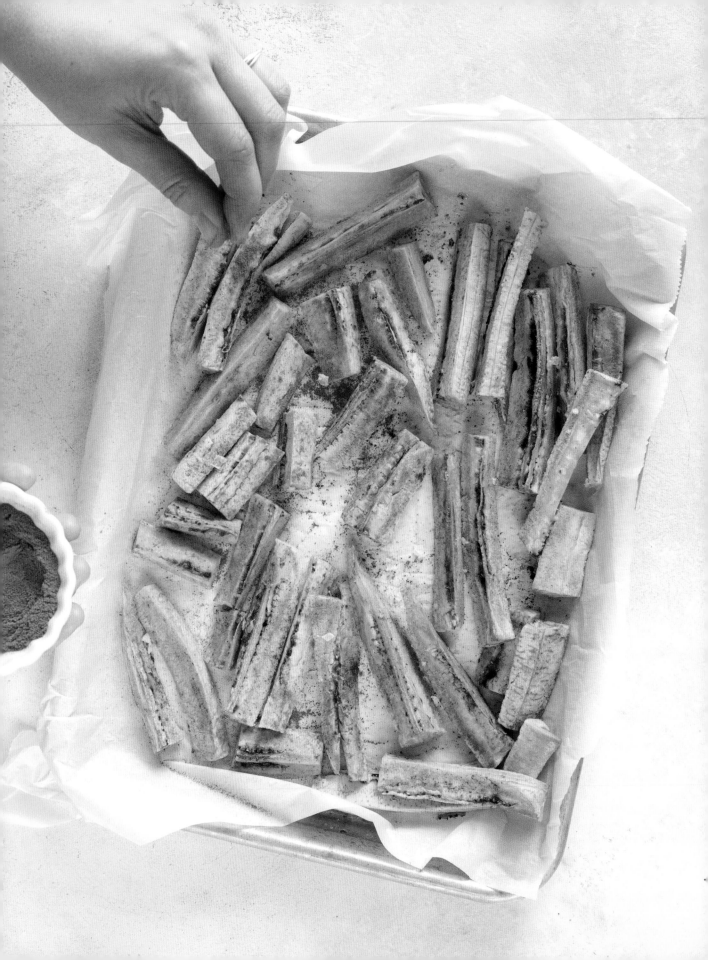

PLÁTANOS MADUROS

MAKES 4 SERVINGS

One of the most common foods in tropical climates, the plantain is incredibly versatile and relatively simple to prepare. Fortunately, at the SOMOS Center in the Dominican Republic, we grow these right outside our kitchen. Larger than bananas, plantains can be consumed whether they are green or yellow and can be found in most grocery stores.

2 ripe plantains (deep yellow to
   dark brown)
1 teaspoon salt
Ground cinnamon

Stovetop

1. Wash the plantains but do not peel them.

2. Cut each plantain (with its peel) into three equal parts.

3. Bring a large pot of water to a boil over medium-high heat. Add the plantains and 1 teaspoon of salt to the boiling water.

4. Boil the plantains until the skins open. At this point, remove the pot from the heat and drain the water.

5. Peel each plantain, then cut into smaller pieces. Season with cinnamon and serve warm.

Oven

1. Preheat oven to 350°F. Line a baking sheet with parchment.

2. Slice through the skin of each plantain and then peel them.

3. Cut each plantain into three equal parts and then cut lengthwise into ¼–½-inch slices.

4. Place the plantain slices on the lined baking sheet. Sprinkle with cinnamon.

5. Bake for 10–15 minutes, turn over plantains, and bake for an additional 5 minutes.

6. Serve warm.

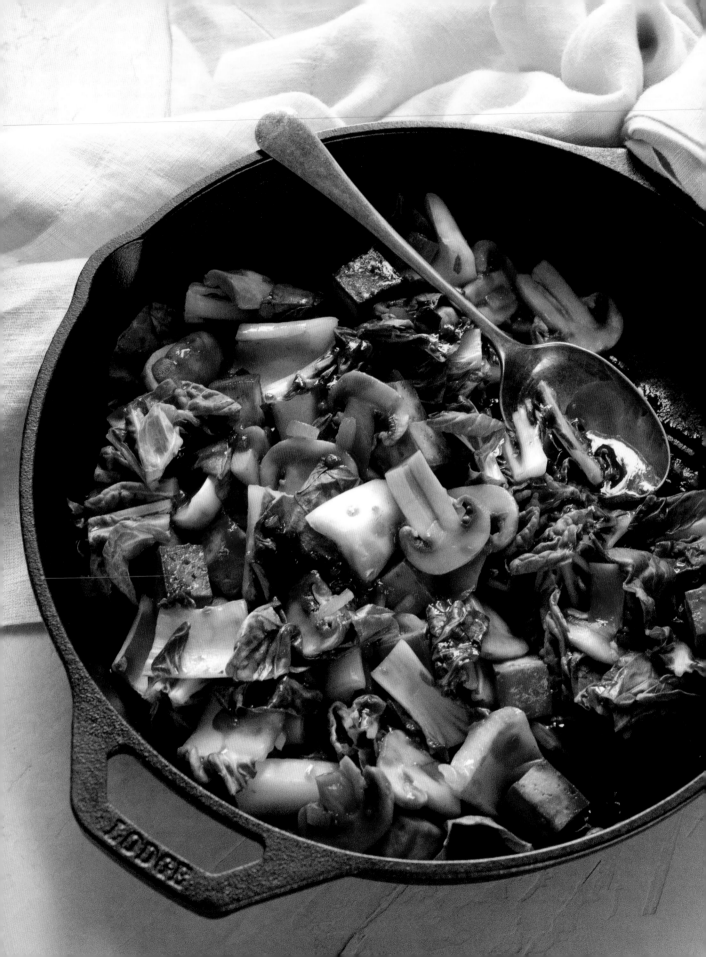

"OYSTER" FLAVORED BOK CHOY WITH MUSHROOMS AND BAKED TOFU

MAKES 3–4 SERVINGS

If there is such a thing as the "Queen of Cooked Greens," that would be my mom. She cooks greens in one form or another nearly every day. And one of her favorite recipes is this flavorful bok choy, which goes well with Fiesta Cornbread (page 44), Creamed Cauliflower (page 254), and Caribbean Moro (page 256).

¼ cup vegetable broth

⅓ cup diced onions

1 pound bok choy, chopped

1 cup sliced mushrooms (baby portobello or button)

1 cup cubed *Baked Tofu* (page 95)

6–8 tablespoons *Vegetarian "Oyster" Sauce* (page 274)

1. In a skillet, combine vegetable broth, onions, and bok choy. Cover and cook over medium heat for 2–3 minutes, until bok choy softens. Add mushrooms and cook for an additional 2–3 minutes.

2. Gently add tofu and 6 tablespoons of sauce. Cook for 2–3 minutes, adding up to 2 tablespoons more sauce if necessary.

3. Serve warm.

PENNY CARROTS

MAKES 4 SERVINGS

When I was younger, my mother made a dish similar to this for Thanksgiving and Christmas. I loved it, especially leftovers, since the carrots were able to marinate for an extra day. But then we stopped making them because of all the oil and sugar. However, I've tweaked the original recipe and it's now back on our holiday menu.

2 medium carrots, cut into ¼-inch-thick rounds

¼ cup diced onions

¼ cup diced green bell peppers

1 medium tomato, pureed

3½ tablespoons apple cider vinegar

3 tablespoons maple syrup

½ teaspoon vegan Worcestershire sauce

1 tablespoon cornstarch

½ teaspoon salt

1. Put the carrots in a small saucepan and cover with water. Cook over medium heat until soft. Drain water from carrots and transfer carrots to a bowl. Add onions and bell peppers.

2. In the same saucepan, whisk together tomato puree, vinegar, maple syrup, Worcestershire sauce, cornstarch, and salt. Cook over medium-high heat, stirring constantly, until it comes to a gentle boil. Remove from heat.

3. Pour the sauce over the vegetables and gently stir until all vegetables are well coated.

4. Cover and refrigerate for 3–4 hours before serving.

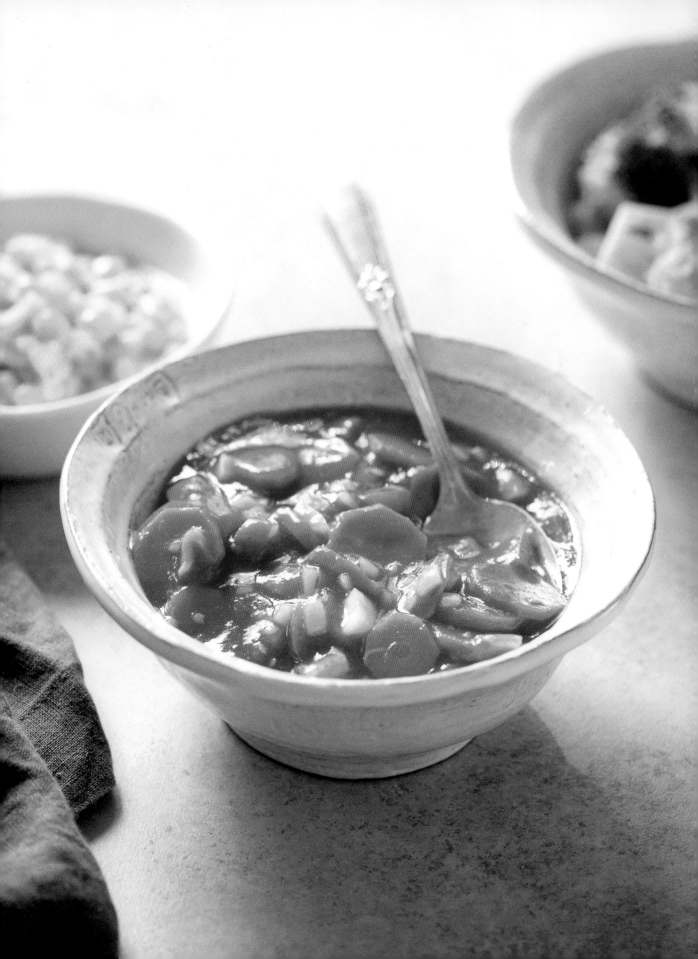

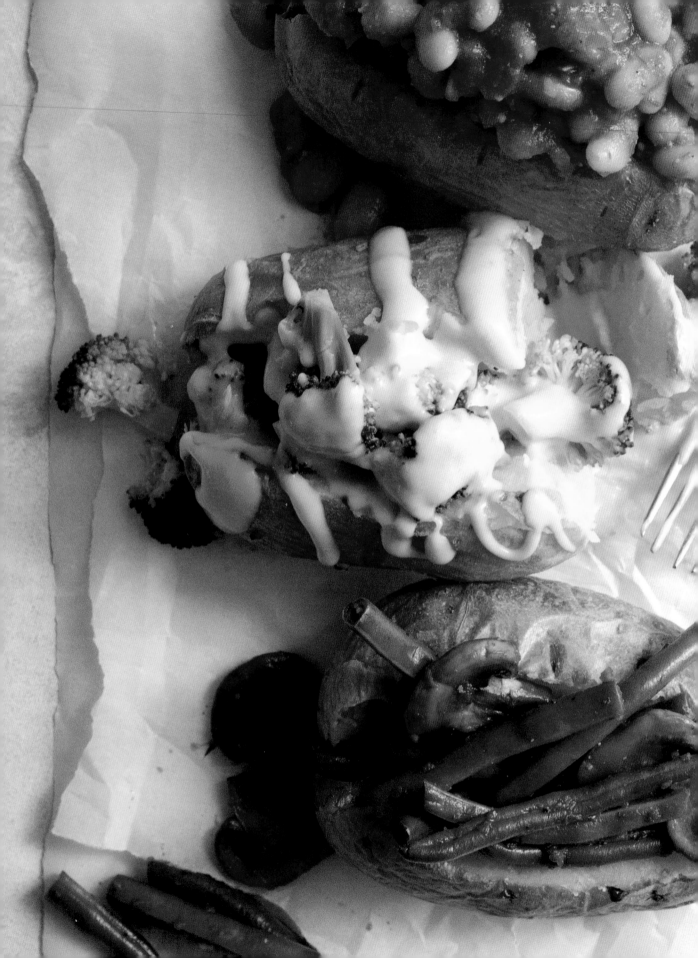

OH-SO-GOOD POTATO BAR

MAKES 4 SERVINGS

Both of my sons, now 24 and 23 years old, were raised on an animal-free diet. When asked by our meat-eating friends what we ate when they were young, I often answer rice and beans or pasta—and of course everything in this book! However, we also ate a lot of potatoes, and one of our favorite meals was "loaded" potatoes. We had these at least once or twice a week, but with different fillings. I often served these potatoes with a large bowl of soup.

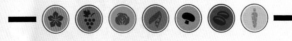

4 large potatoes, baked

Optional Toppings
Baked Beans (page 250)
Coleslaws (pages 100–101)
Fasolia (page 265)
Steamed broccoli with *Creamy Dijon Sauce* (page 274)
Mushroom Gravy (page 202)

SAVORY GOODNESS: SAUCES FOR STEAMED VEGETABLES

In our home, we have fresh vegetables, lightly cooked (preferably steamed), with every meal. If I have one of these sauces on hand, I'll drizzle it on the vegetables, especially if I'm serving it with a portion of brown rice.

CREAMY DIJON SAUCE

(goes well with potatoes and eggplant)

MAKES ABOUT 1 CUP

⅓ cup raw cashews

½ cup water

½ teaspoon Dijon mustard

1 tablespoon nutritional yeast

1 tablespoon white miso

Blend all ingredients in a food processor until smooth.

VEGETARIAN "OYSTER" SAUCE

(goes well with broccoli, bell peppers, onions, and carrots)

MAKES ABOUT 1 CUP

½ cup vegetable broth

½ cup reduced-sodium soy sauce

¼ cup maple syrup

2 tablespoons rice vinegar

4 garlic cloves, minced

1 tablespoon grated fresh ginger

1 tablespoon cornstarch mixed with 1 tablespoon water

⅛ teaspoon Sriracha sauce (optional)

Combine all ingredients in a saucepan and cook over medium-high heat until mixture thickens.

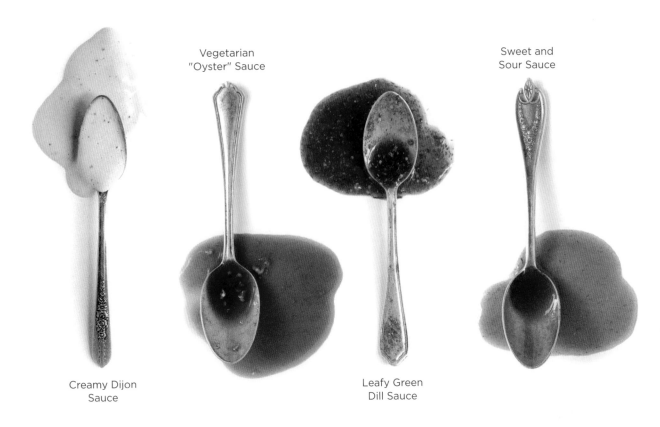

Vegetarian "Oyster" Sauce

Sweet and Sour Sauce

Creamy Dijon Sauce

Leafy Green Dill Sauce

LEAFY GREEN DILL SAUCE

(goes well with kale, collards, spinach, and other greens)

MAKES ABOUT 1 CUP

¼ cup lemon juice

¼ cup reduced-sodium soy sauce

1 tablespoon Dijon mustard

1 teaspoon dried dill

1 teaspoon cornstarch mixed with 2 tablespoons water

Combine all ingredients in a saucepan and cook over medium-high heat until mixture thickens.

SWEET AND SOUR SAUCE

(goes well with broccoli, bell peppers, onions, and carrots)

MAKES ABOUT 1 CUP

5 tablespoons apple cider vinegar

¼ cup reduced-sodium soy sauce

¼ cup water

2 tablespoons orange juice

2 tablespoons ketchup

¼ cup raw cane sugar

1 tablespoon cornstarch or arrowroot powder

Combine all ingredients in a saucepan and cook over medium heat until mixture thickens.

SUSHI GINGER EDAMAME

MAKES 4 SERVINGS

I love sushi, especially with sweet pickled ginger, or gari. Made from young ginger root and marinated in a solution of sugar and vinegar, gari is meant to be eaten between different pieces of sushi. However, I love it not only to cleanse my palate, but also served with rice and edamame, giving it the perfect ginger flavor.

2 cups chopped broccoli, steamed

1 cup edamame, cooked

¼ cup thinly sliced green onions

¼ cup sliced gari (sushi ginger), plus more to taste

1 tablespoon reduced-sodium soy sauce, plus more to taste

1 tablespoon rice wine vinegar

1 cup cooked brown rice

Stir together all ingredients, taste, and if needed, add additional gari or soy sauce. Enjoy!

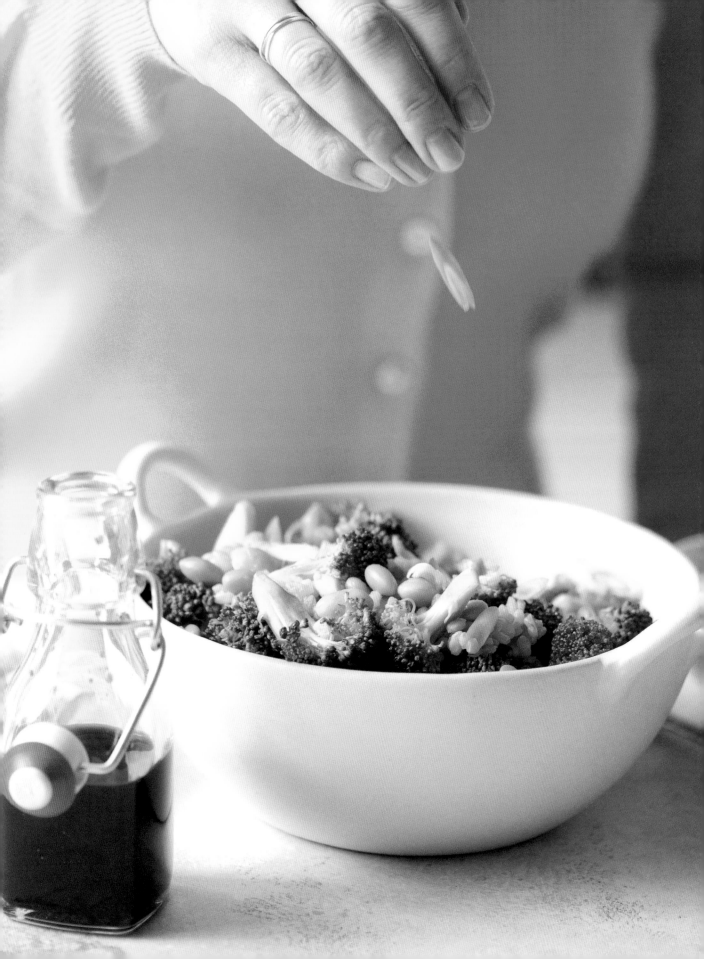

SWEET POTATOES AND KALE

MAKES 4–5 SERVINGS

The first time I cooked kale, I didn't like it. But now I love it, and I buy it at least twice a week! What I've learned is that you need to make the perfect sauce. So in this recipe, I've used a lemon mustard sauce and then added a touch of sweetness from diced sweet potatoes.

2 sweet potatoes, peeled and diced (about 4 cups)

2 tablespoons vegetable broth

¼ cup diced onion

1 bunch kale, chopped (6–7 cups)

6–8 tablespoons *Leafy Green Dill Sauce* (page 275)

1. Put potatoes in a pot and cover with water. Cook over medium-high heat until potatoes are soft but not mushy. Drain.

2. Combine vegetable broth, onion, and kale in a medium-size skillet. Cover and cook over medium-high heat for 3–5 minutes, until kale softens.

3. Add potatoes to skillet.

4. Gently stir in 6 tablespoons of dill sauce. Cook for 2–3 minutes, adding up to 2 tablespoons more sauce if necessary.

5. Serve warm.

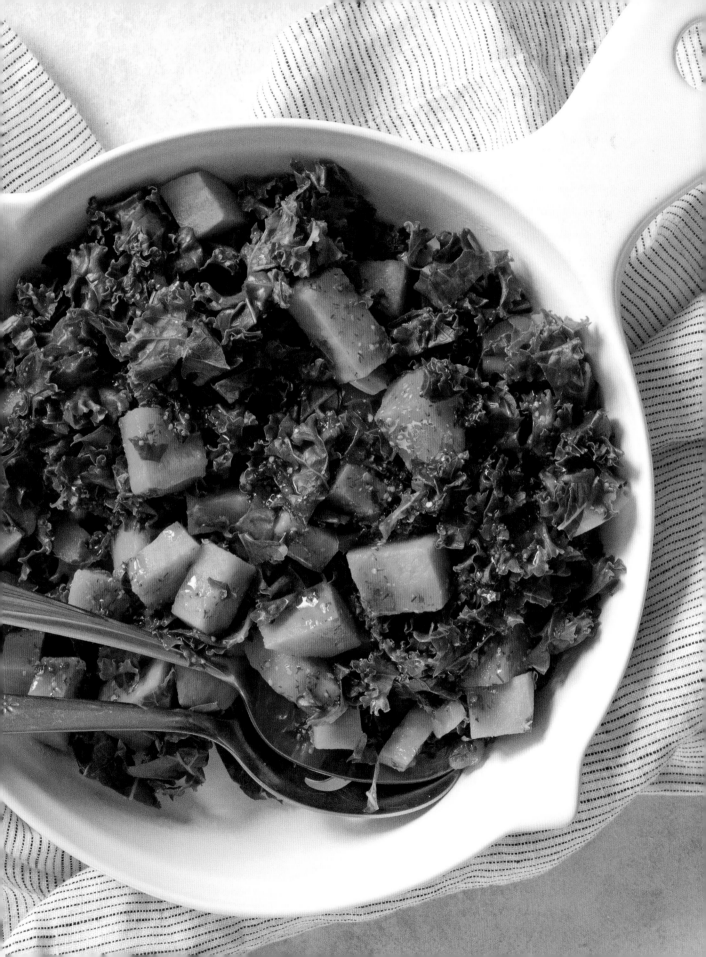

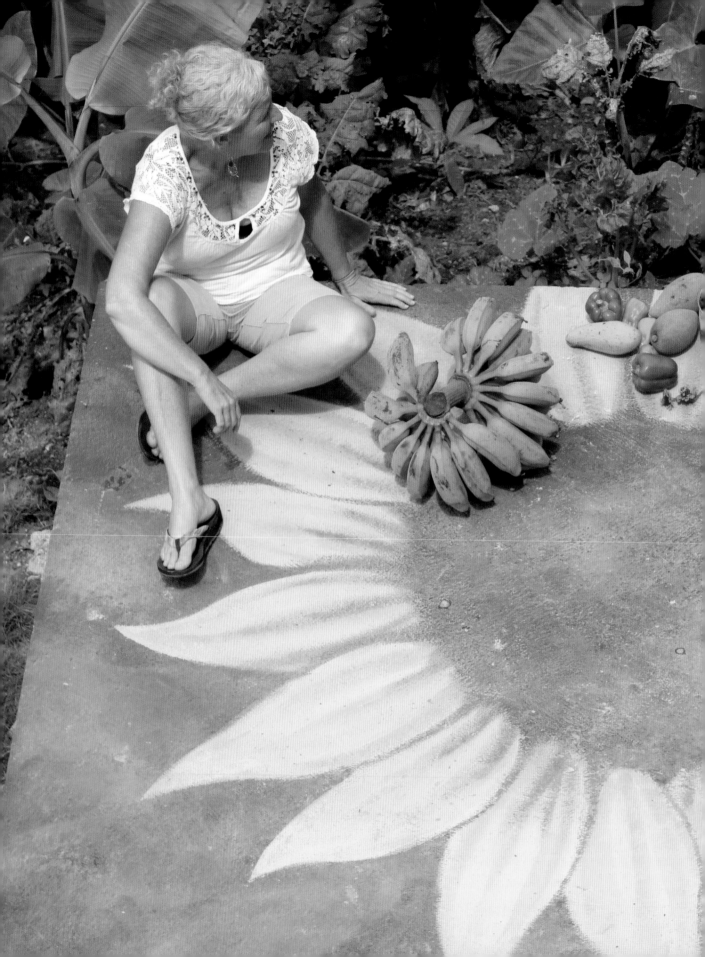

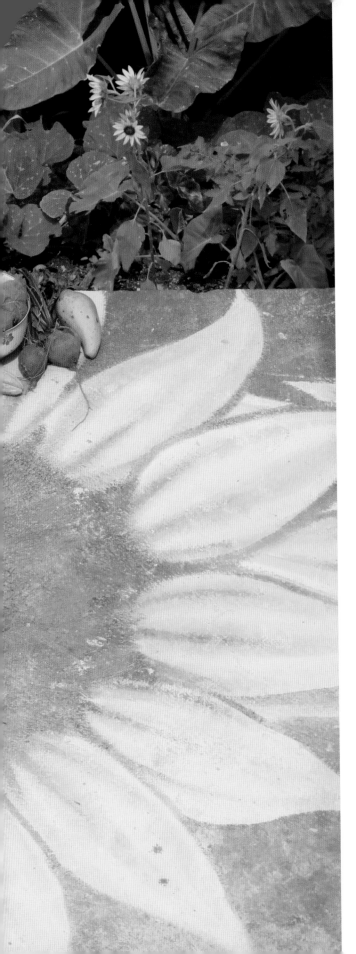

DESERTS

AMAZINGLY DELICIOUS DATE FRUIT PIE

MAKES 6 SERVINGS

The first time I had a no-bake pie crust, I was visiting a friend in Florida. We had it at a local vegetarian festival, and I knew I had to have it again. So that evening I made my own version and loaded it with fresh fruit. Not surprisingly, this became one of my family's favorites. If I don't have Medjool dates on hand, dried plums (prunes) are just as good.

3–4 cups fresh fruit (sliced strawberries, blackberries, blueberries, sliced mangos, sliced kiwis, or similar)

1 *No-Bake Date Crust* (page 304)

1. Arrange fruit on top of chilled pie crust.
2. Chill for 1 hour before serving.

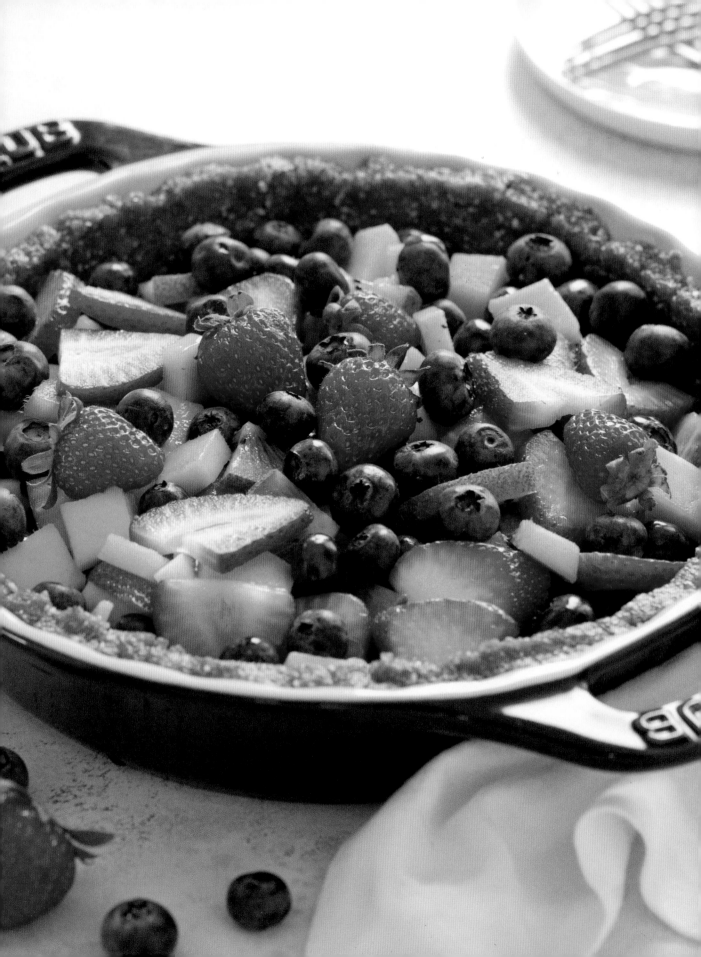

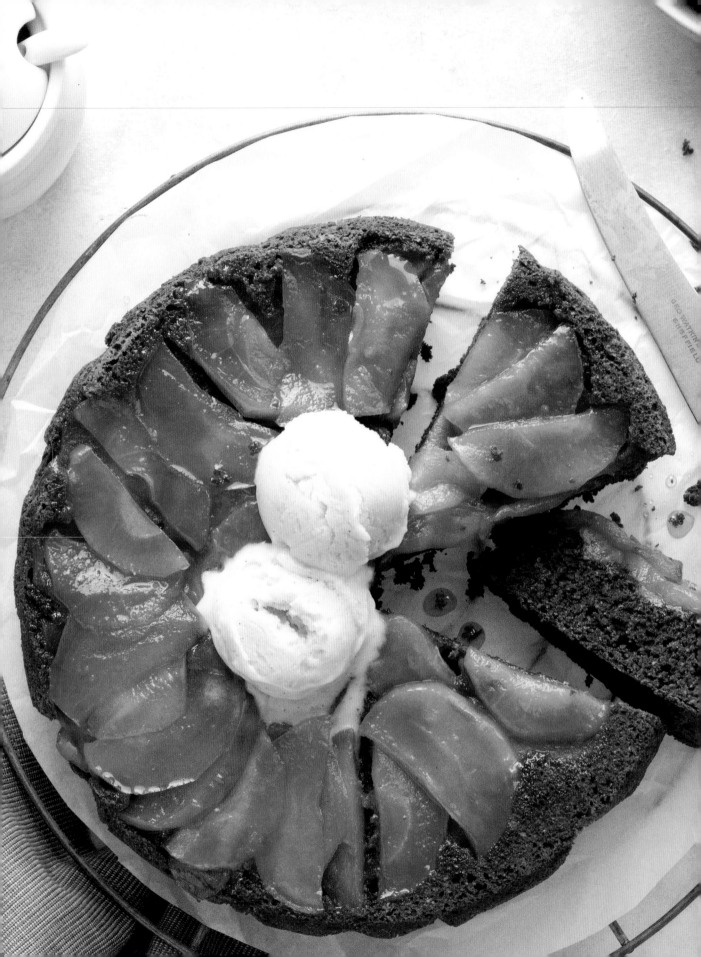

APPLE GINGERBREAD UPSIDE-DOWN CAKE

MAKES 6 SERVINGS

If you like molasses, you'll love this cake. It's especially good with baked apples and a scoop of Vanilla Cream (page 297). Just make sure to use light molasses, which comes from the first boiling of the sugar, rather than blackstrap or dark molasses, which has a much more intense flavor.

3 medium apples, peeled, cored, and sliced

¼ cup maple syrup

1½ cups whole wheat pastry flour

1 teaspoon baking soda

½ teaspoon ground cinnamon

½ teaspoon ground ginger

⅛ teaspoon salt

½ cup hot water

½ cup molasses

¼ cup applesauce

1 recipe *Vanilla Cream* (page 297), for serving (optional)

1. Preheat oven to 350°F.

2. Place apples and maple syrup in a medium-size pan. Cover and cook over medium heat for 4–5 minutes, until apples are slightly soft. Remove from heat.

3. In a small bowl, whisk together flour, baking soda, cinnamon, ginger, and salt.

4. In a separate bowl, whisk together hot water, molasses, and applesauce. Fold into dry ingredients.

5. Spread cooked apples evenly on the bottom of a 8 × 8-inch nonstick baking dish. Pour batter over apples.

6. Bake for 35–40 minutes, until a toothpick inserted in the center comes out clean.

7. While cake is still warm, place a serving plate over baking dish and carefully flip the cake onto the plate. Serve warm, topped with vanilla cream if desired.

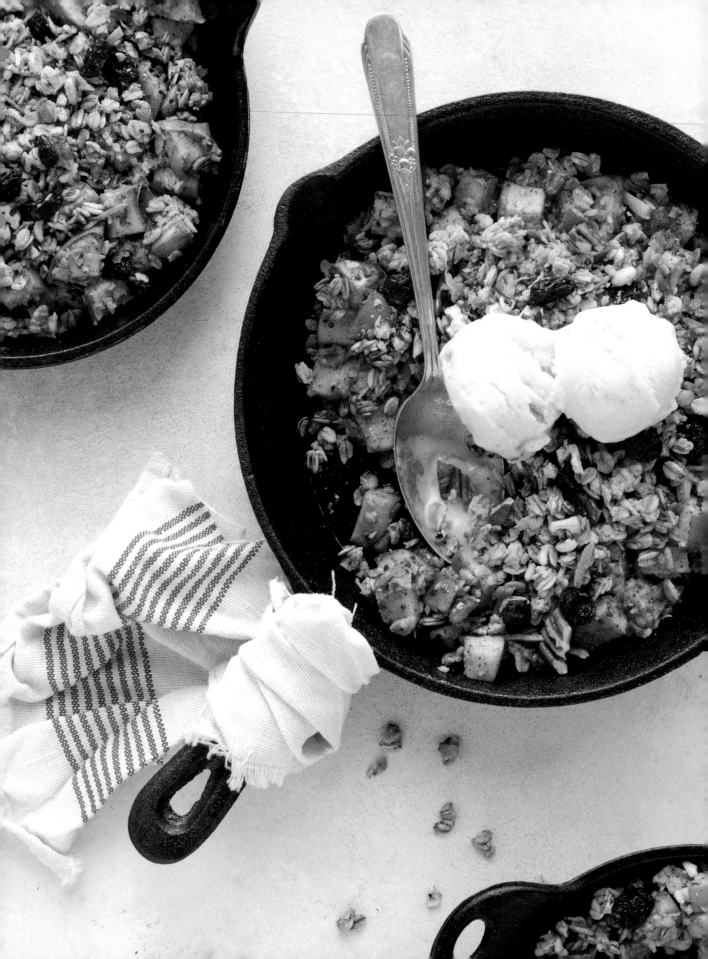

APPLE PIE CRISP

MAKES 4 SERVINGS

When making apple deserts, the trick is choosing the right apple. I like to cook with McIntosh apples. They bake quickly and taste absolutely delicious. If you're using a sweeter apple (Red Delicious or Gala), you will need to cook the crisp for an additional 20 minutes.

4 cups peeled and diced apples
¼ cup apple juice concentrate
½ teaspoon ground cinnamon
½ teaspoon ground nutmeg
1½ cups granola or *Nature's Granola* **(page 74)**

1. Preheat oven to 350°F.

2. In an 8 × 8-inch nonstick baking dish, stir together apples, apple juice concentrate, cinnamon, nutmeg, and ¾ cup of granola. Spread evenly. Sprinkle remaining granola on top.

3. Cover with aluminum foil and bake for 35–40 minutes. Serve warm.

CHOCOLATE BROWNIE BIRTHDAY CAKE

MAKES 6–8 SERVINGS

If you are big fan of brownies, you'll love this cake. The creamy sweet potato icing is something I learned from my good friend Chef Del Sroufe, and it is a wonderful addition to this cake. I serve it with one of my favorite frozen delights—Chocolate Cravings (page 296).

Cake

2 cups whole wheat flour

¾ cup raw cane sugar

⅓ cup cocoa powder

1 teaspoon baking powder

½ teaspoon baking soda

1½ cups unsweetened nondairy milk (rice, soy, almond, etc.)

⅓ cup applesauce

1 teaspoon vanilla extract

Chocolate Frosting

½ cup diced cooked sweet potatoes

¼ cup Medjool dates

3 tablespoons cocoa powder

2 cups raspberries

1 recipe *Chocolate Cravings* (page 296)

1. Preheat oven to 350°F. Line two round cake pans with parchment.

2. In a large bowl, whisk together flour, sugar, cocoa, baking powder, and baking soda.

3. In a separate bowl, whisk together milk, applesauce, and vanilla. Fold into dry mixture.

4. Divide batter between lined cake pans. Bake for 20–25 minutes, until a toothpick inserted in the center comes out clean. Cool on wire racks.

5. While cake is baking, prepare frosting by blending sweet potatoes, dates, and cocoa powder in a food processor until smooth.

6. When cakes are cool, spread icing on the tops of both cakes. Place raspberries on top of one cake and then layer with the second cake.

7. Serve topped with chocolate cravings.

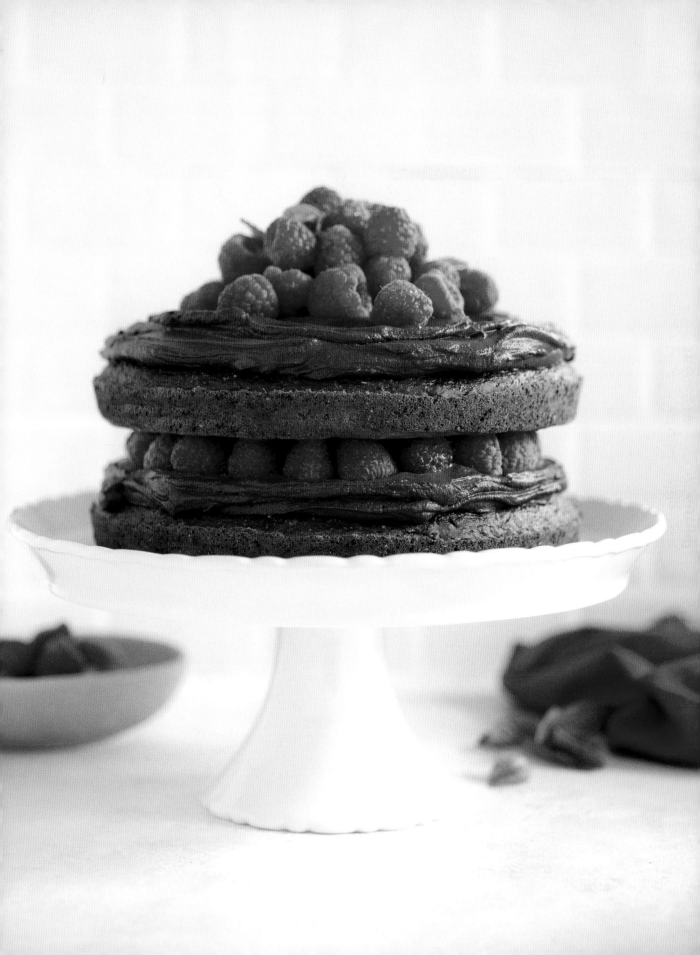

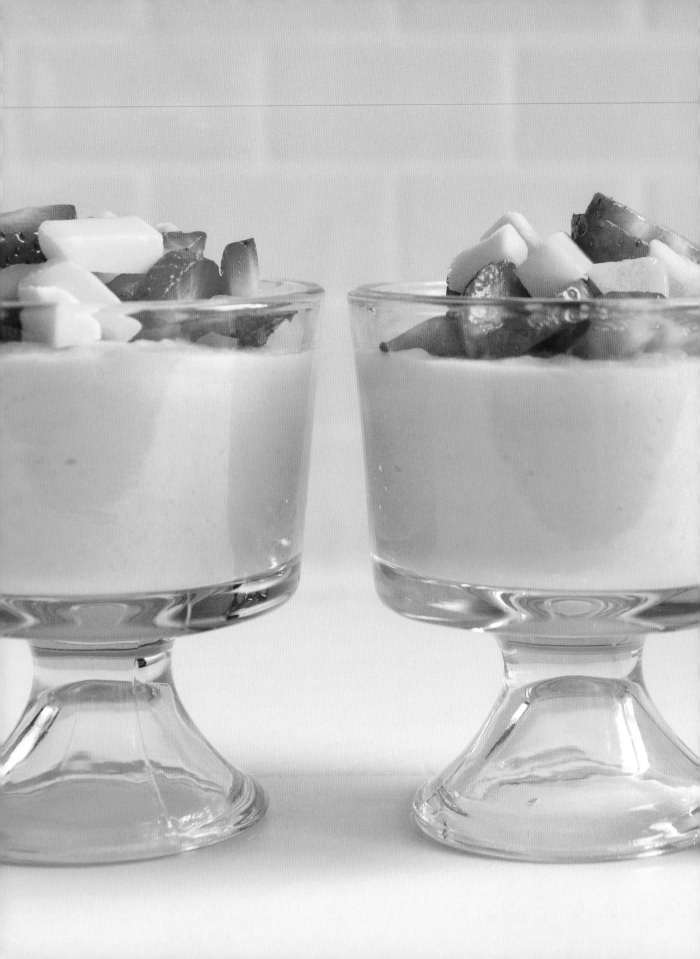

COCONUT MANGO PUDDING

MAKES 3–4 SERVINGS

I love mangos, especially with a bit of lime. There are some 400 varieties of mangos, with some being sweeter than others, so I adjust the amount of sweetener that I add depending on the type of mango and ripeness. In some cases, I skip the sugar altogether.

1 (13½-ounce) can unsweetened coconut milk

1 cup pureed mango

1–4 tablespoons raw cane sugar

¼ cup unsweetened nondairy milk (rice, soy, almond, etc.) mixed with 2 tablespoons cornstarch

1 teaspoon lime juice

Sliced mangos and strawberries, for topping

1. Combine coconut milk, mango puree, and cane sugar in a medium-size sauce pan. Bring to a boil over medium-high heat.

2. Stir in milk with cornstarch and lime juice. Continue boiling until mixture becomes thick, 2–3 minutes. Remove from heat.

3. Pour into serving dishes and refrigerate until thickened.

4. Garnish with mangos and strawberries.

CREAMY CHOCOLATE PIE

MAKES 6–8 SERVINGS

I love chocolate, and one of the wonderful bonuses of living in the Dominican Republic is that I have cocoa trees growing on my land, allowing me to stock my shelves with balls of cocoa. One of the things I love to make with these cocoa balls is this chocolate pudding pie, using a graham cracker crust and fresh fruit.

1 recipe *Sweet Graham Crust* (page 305)

3 tablespoons cocoa powder

¼ cup raw cane sugar

1 cup unsweetened nondairy milk (rice, soy, almond, etc.)

6 tablespoons cornstarch mixed with 1 cup unsweetened nondairy milk (rice, soy, almond, etc.)

½ cup vegan chocolate chips

1 cup sliced strawberries or bananas

¼ cup crushed slivered almonds

1. Preheat oven to 350°F.

2. Bake pie crust for 12–15 minutes.

3. Meanwhile, in a saucepan, combine cocoa, sugar, and milk. Bring to a boil over medium-high heat. Add cornstarch mixture. Reduce heat and simmer gently for 3–5 minutes, stirring constantly, until mixture thickens. Add chocolate chips and stir until chips melt.

4. Layer sliced fruit in bottom of baked pie crust. Pour chocolate mixture over fruit and sprinkle with almonds.

5. Refrigerate until firm, 3–4 hours.

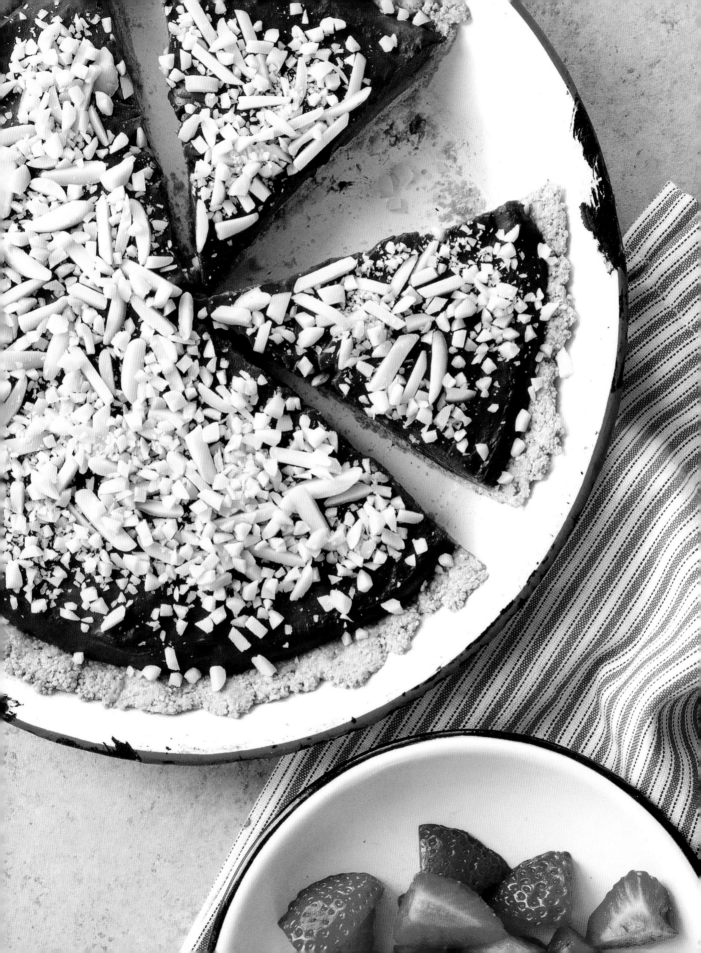

EVERY NIGHT FROZEN DELIGHTS

Super easy and so satisfying, these frozen treats hit the spot for that late-night sweet craving. Just make sure you have a few bags of frozen bananas on hand—and remember, the riper the bananas, the sweeter the cream. So if you have some super ripe bananas, peel them and place them in a resealable plastic bag in the freezer.

CHOCOLATE CRAVINGS

MAKES 2 SERVINGS

3 frozen bananas

1 cup unsweetened nondairy milk (rice, soy, almond, etc.)

2–3 tablespoons cocoa powder

Blend all ingredients in a food processor until smooth. If needed, add more milk.

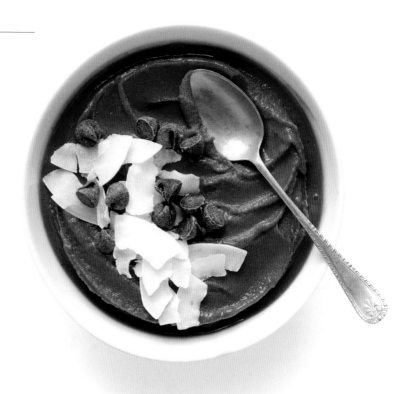

PEANUT BUTTER CREAM

MAKES 2 SERVINGS

3 frozen bananas

1 cup unsweetened nondairy milk (rice, soy, almond, etc.)

3-4 tablespoons natural peanut butter

Blend all ingredients in a food processor until smooth. If needed, add more milk.

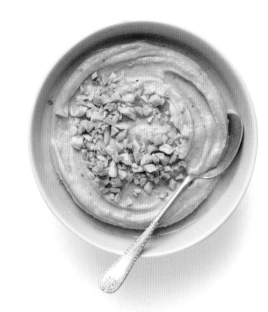

VANILLA CREAM

MAKES 2 SERVINGS

3 frozen bananas

1 cup unsweetened nondairy milk (rice, soy, almond, etc.)

1 teaspoon vanilla extract

Blend all ingredients in a food processor until smooth. If needed, add more milk.

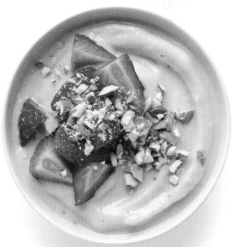

COOL MINT

MAKES 2 SERVINGS

3 frozen bananas

1 cup unsweetened nondairy milk (rice, soy, almond, etc.)

2 tablespoons chopped fresh mint or 1 teaspoon mint extract

Blend all ingredients in a food processor until smooth. If needed, add more milk.

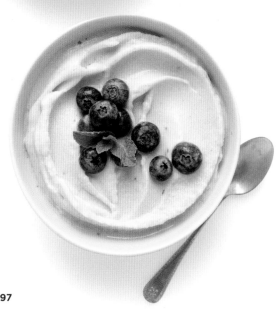

NO-BAKE CHOCOLATE OATMEAL DROPS

MAKES 12 COOKIES

I used to love opening my school lunch box to find these cookies—my all-time favorites! Not surprisingly, they were also a hit with my sons. And as the one packing their lunch boxes, I loved the ease of making this treat—5 minutes to prep and 15 minutes to chill in the freezer.

- 1 cup unsweetened nondairy milk (rice, soy, almond, etc.)
- ½ cup natural peanut butter
- ⅓ cup raw cane sugar
- 3 tablespoons cocoa powder
- 2 cups rolled oats

1. In a saucepan, cook milk, peanut butter, and sugar over medium-high heat, stirring constantly, until peanut butter dissolves.

2. Add cocoa powder and continue to stir. Add oats, stir, and cook for 1–2 minutes.

3. Remove from heat and divide into 12 balls on a baking sheet. Press with a spoon until flat. Refrigerate or freeze before serving.

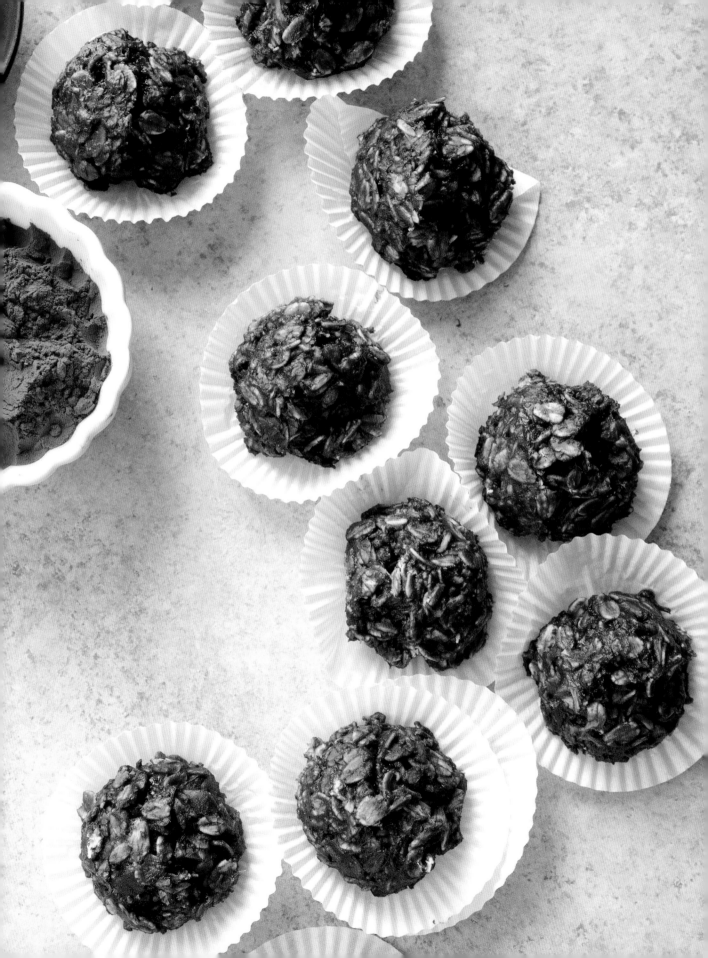

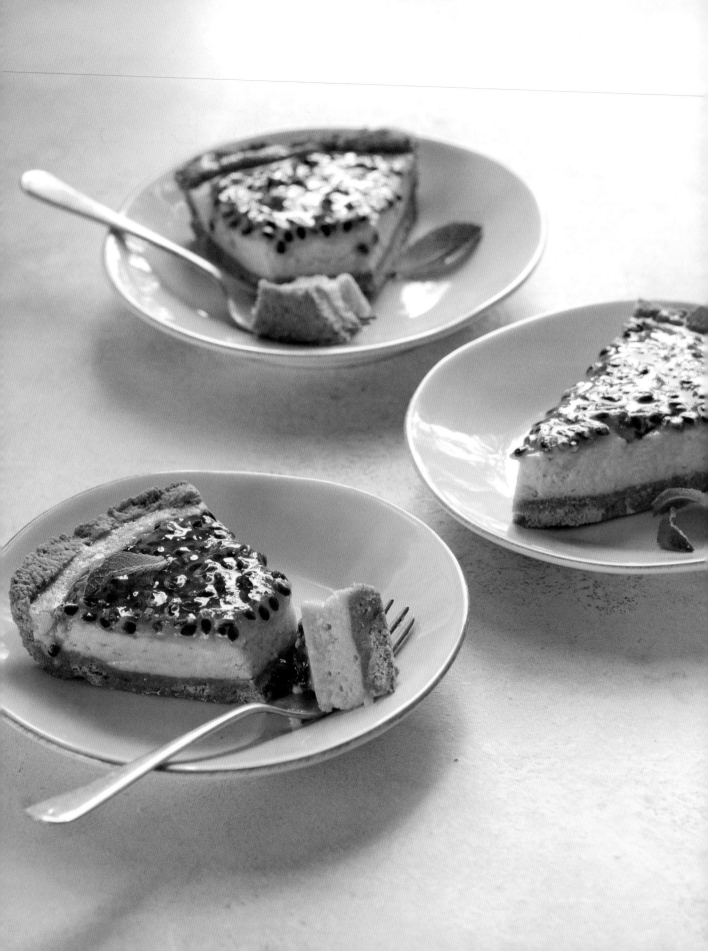

PASSION FRUIT BLISS OR BLACK CHERRY CHEESE(LESS) CAKE DELIGHT

MAKES 6 SERVINGS

This version of the traditional cheesecake is not only free of dairy and processed oil, but it's delicious, simple, and can be topped with many different fruit combinations. I've listed a couple of my favorites, with passion fruit being at the top of my list!

Filling
12 ounces silken tofu
¼ cup raw cashews
¼ cup raw cane sugar
2 tablespoons cornstarch
⅛ teaspoon salt
½ cup unsweetened nondairy milk (soy or almond)
4 teaspoons lemon juice

1 recipe *Sweet Graham Crust* (page 305)

Topping Option 1: Passion Fruit Bliss
½ cup passion fruit seeds
¼ cup raw cane sugar

Topping Option 2: Glazed Sweet Black Cherries
1½ cups sweet black cherries, pitted
¼ cup water
1 tablespoon cornstarch
1 tablespoon raw cane sugar

1. Combine all filling ingredients in a medium saucepan and simmer for 2–3 minutes, stirring constantly, until it becomes slightly thick.

2. Preheat oven to 350°F.

3. In a food processor, puree filling until creamy.

4. Spread mixture in pie crust and bake for 40–45 minutes.

5. While cake is baking, prepare your choice of fruit topping. Combine all ingredients in a medium saucepan and simmer for 2–3 minutes, stirring constantly, until mixture becomes slightly thick. (For Glazed Sweet Black Cherries, blend the cornstarch and sugar before adding it to the mixture.)

6. Once cake is baked and cooled, spread fruit topping evenly on top. Refrigerate for 1–2 hours before serving.

PEANUT BUTTER BARS

MAKES 6–7 SERVINGS

During the holidays, this is one of my favorite treats to make. Sometimes I roll the graham cracker mixture into balls and then dip them into the chocolate mixture. Not only do family and friends love them, but it's nice to have others around to help eat them. Otherwise, I'll eat the entire pan before the day ends!

1 cup ground low-fat graham crackers

¼ cup finely chopped walnuts

½ cup unsweetened shredded coconut

⅓ cup natural peanut butter

¼ cup unsweetened nondairy milk (rice, soy, almond, etc.), plus more as needed

Chocolate Topping

1 cup vegan chocolate chips

5 tablespoons unsweetened nondairy milk (rice, soy, almond, etc.)

1. In a large bowl, combine graham cracker crumbs, walnuts, coconut, and peanut butter. Stir well.

2. Slowly add milk and mix. If mixture does not hold together, continue adding additional milk until all ingredients stick together. However, don't make it too soft; use your hands if necessary.

3. Spread mixture into a 9 × 9-inch nonstick baking dish.

4. To make chocolate topping, melt chocolate chips and nondairy milk in a small saucepan over medium heat. Stir until smooth.

5. Spread chocolate mixture on top of peanut butter mixture. Refrigerate for 2–3 hours, until hardened. Cut into squares and enjoy!

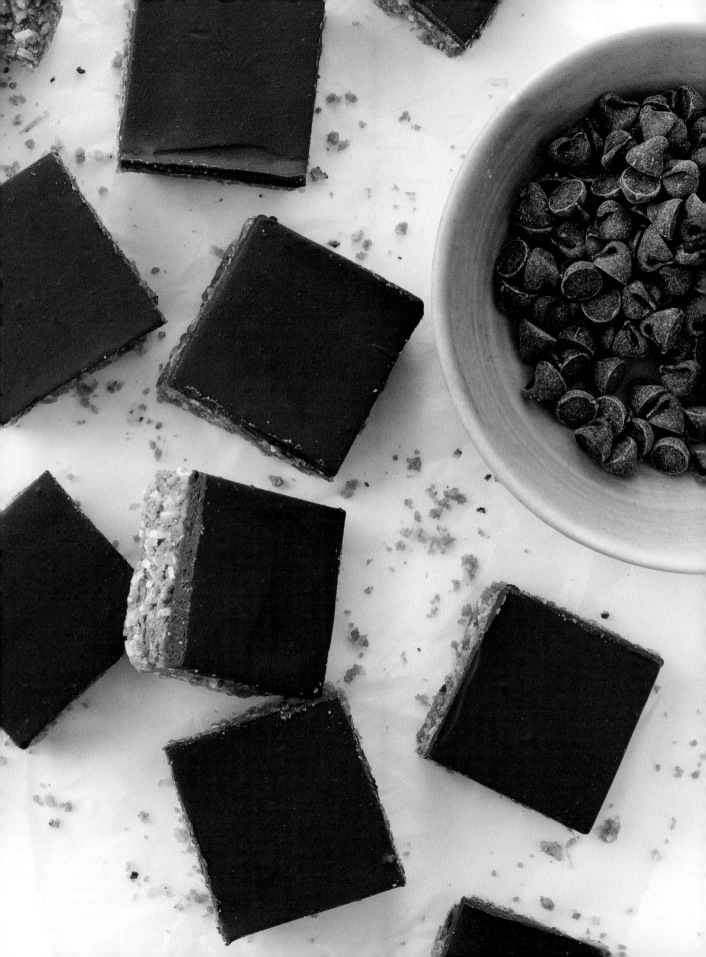

PIE CRUSTS

It takes some creativity to make a flaky pie crust with no added oil. With the traditional graham cracker crust, I replace the butter with applesauce, and for a no-bake pie crust, I use dried fruit and nuts. For pies that need to be baked, like pumpkin and sweet potato pies, I like to use the Cocoa Powder Crust.

NO-BAKE DATE CRUST

MAKES 1 PIE CRUST

1 cup Medjool dates or dried plums (prunes)

1 cup walnuts or pecans

1 teaspoon vanilla extract

½ cup unsweetened shredded coconut

½ teaspoon ground cinnamon

1. Blend all ingredients in a food processor at high speed until a ball forms.

2. Press into a nonstick pie pan and chill until ready to use.

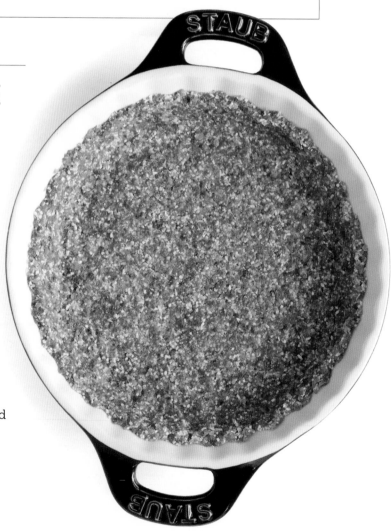

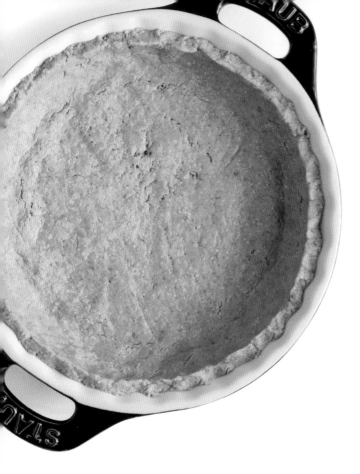

SWEET GRAHAM CRUST

MAKES 1 PIE CRUST

1½ cups ground low-fat graham crackers
6–7 tablespoons applesauce

1. Blend graham cracker crumbs and 6 tablespoons of applesauce in a food processor until a ball forms. If mixture is dry, add an additional tablespoon of applesauce.

2. Press into a nonstick pie pan.

COCOA POWDER CRUST

MAKES 1 PIE CRUST

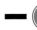

1 cup rolled oats
8 Medjool dates, pitted
½ cup walnuts
6–7 tablespoons applesauce
2 tablespoons maple syrup
2 tablespoons cocoa powder

1. Blend oats in a food processor. Add dates, walnuts, 6 tablespoons of applesauce, maple syrup, and cocoa powder and blend until a soft ball forms. If mixture is dry, add an additional tablespoon of applesauce.

2. Press into a nonstick pie pan.

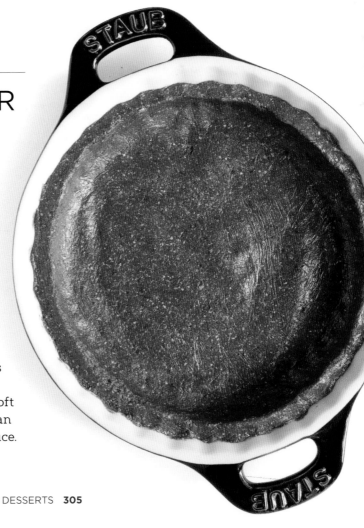

PINEAPPLE CHERRY COBBLER

MAKES 6 SERVINGS

My mother first learned how to make this family favorite from a local barber. However, he used a cake mix and added melted butter to the top. We loved his original version, but we have since modified the recipe, making our own oat flour mixture and replacing the melted butter with pineapple juice. It's especially good topped with Vanilla Cream (page 297).

1 (20-ounce) can crushed pineapple in juice

1 (14½-ounce) can pitted tart cherries, drained

½ cup unsweetened shredded coconut (optional)

2 cups rolled oats

½ cup raw cane sugar

½ teaspoon ground ginger

½ cup pineapple juice

1. Preheat oven to 350°F.

2. In an 8 × 8-inch nonstick baking dish, spread crushed pineapple and juice, sour cherries, and coconut (if using).

3. Lightly pulse oats in a food processor to make oat flour. Transfer to a bowl and add cane sugar and ground ginger. Spread oat mixture on top of fruit. Drizzle pineapple juice on top of oats.

4. Bake for 30–35 minutes. Serve warm.

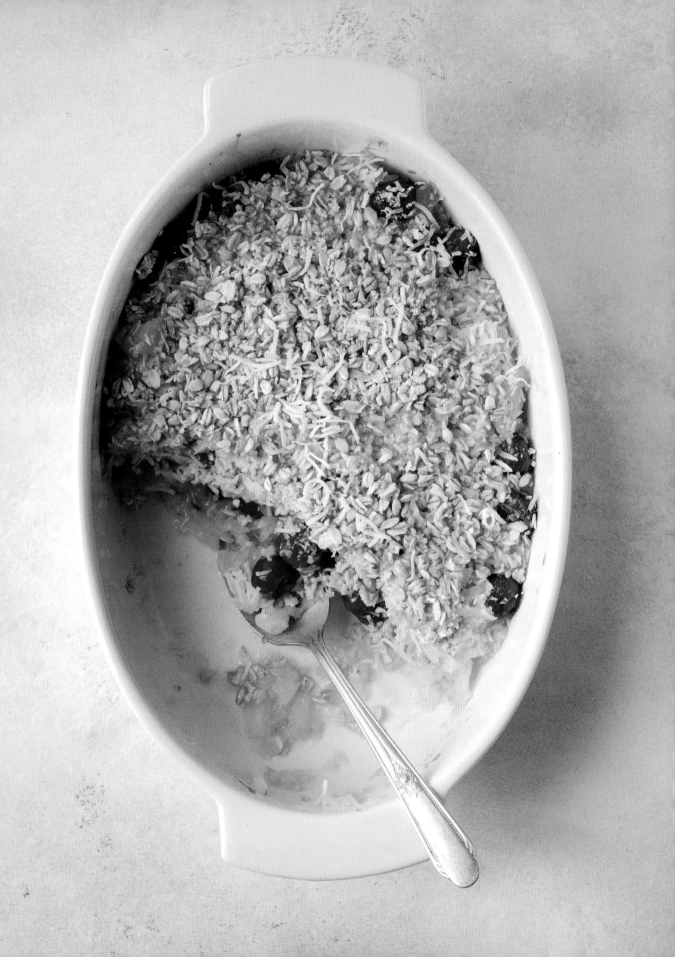

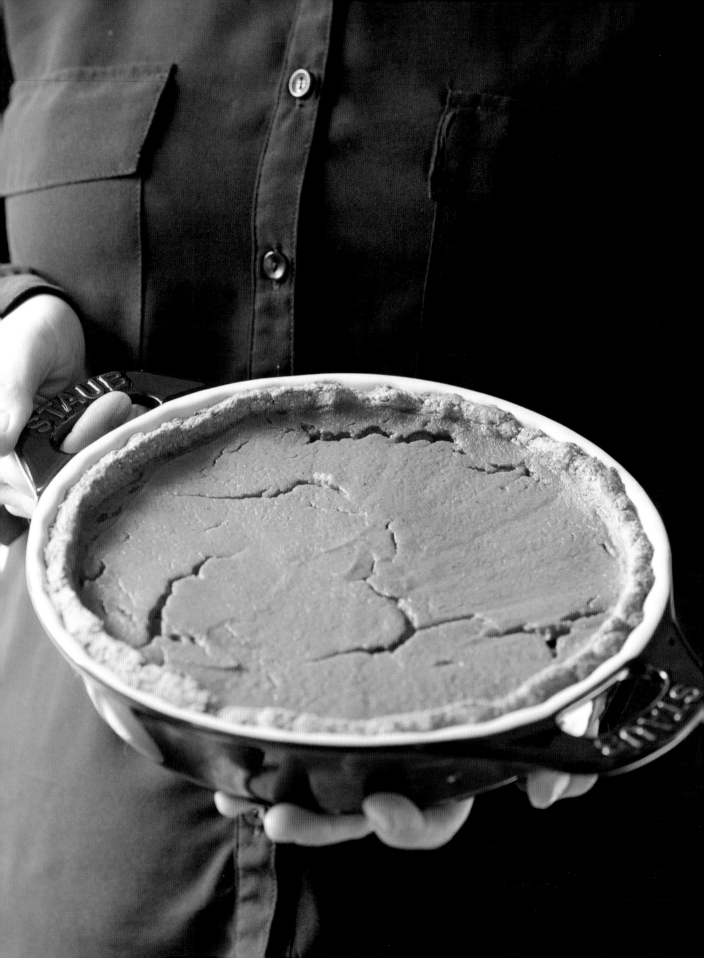

QUICK AND EASY PUMPKIN PIE

MAKES 1 PIE

This simple, flavorful pumpkin pie can be made with either the Sweet Graham Crust (page 305) or the Cocoa Powder Crust (page 305). When in the Dominican Republic, I replace the pumpkin with an orange squash called *auyama*.

1¾ cups canned pumpkin puree

⅔ cup unsweetened nondairy milk (soy or almond)

½ cup raw cane sugar

2 tablespoons arrowroot powder

1 teaspoon ground cinnamon

¼ teaspoon ground nutmeg

¼ teaspoon ground ginger

1 recipe *Cocoa Powder Crust* (page 305) or 1 recipe *Sweet Graham Crust* (page 305)

1. Preheat oven to 350°F.

2. In a food processor, blend pumpkin puree, milk, sugar, arrowroot, cinnamon, nutmeg, and ginger until smooth and creamy.

3. Pour into pie crust.

4. Bake for approximately 1 hour. The pie should be firm, with a couple of open cracks across the top. Let it cool and set for about 5 hours before serving.

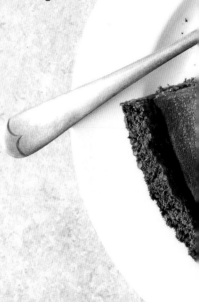

REESE'S PEANUT BUTTER PIE

MAKES 1 PIE

I love the combination of peanut butter and chocolate, and this pie satisfies that craving every time. Because it's so rich, I make it only on special occasions and I limit myself to a small slice. But what's nice about this pie is that it's even better the next day!

1 cup sweet potato puree
½ cup canned coconut milk
½ cup natural peanut butter
¼ cup maple syrup
½–¾ cup vegan chocolate chips
1 recipe *Cocoa Powder Crust* (page 305)

1. Preheat oven to 350°F.

2. In a food processor, blend sweet potato puree, milk, peanut butter, and maple syrup until smooth.

3. Place chocolate chips in bottom of pie crust, then top with blended sweet potato mixture.

4. Bake for 45 minutes, until pie is golden brown and firm.

5. Refrigerate for 1–2 hours before serving.

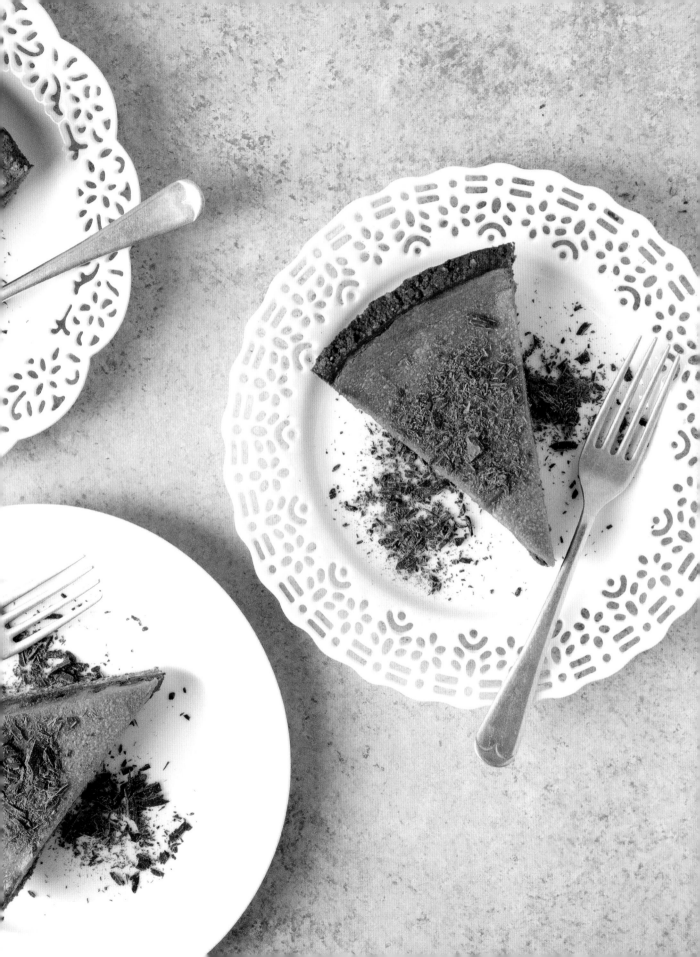

SUMMERTIME NO-BAKE FRUIT PIES

MAKES 8 SERVINGS

This is our go-to pie. We make it all the time, especially during the summer months when we can pick our own berries and fruit. Even for birthday dinners, this is our most requested pie. I often choose strawberry for my birthday, and my younger son selects blueberry.

1 recipe *Sweet Graham Crust* (page 305)
2½ cups berries or sliced fruit (such as peaches)
¾ cups water
⅓ cup raw cane sugar
2 tablespoons cornstarch

1. Preheat oven to 350°F.
2. Bake pie crust for 8–10 minutes.
3. Layer 1½ cups of sliced fresh fruit in pie crust.
4. In a medium saucepan, combine remaining sliced fruit with water and boil over medium heat until fruit begins to dissolve. Whisk together sugar and cornstarch and stir into boiling mixture. Boil, stirring constantly, for 3–4 minutes, until mixture thickens.
5. Pour mixture over fresh fruit in pie crust.
6. Refrigerate 2–3 hours before serving.

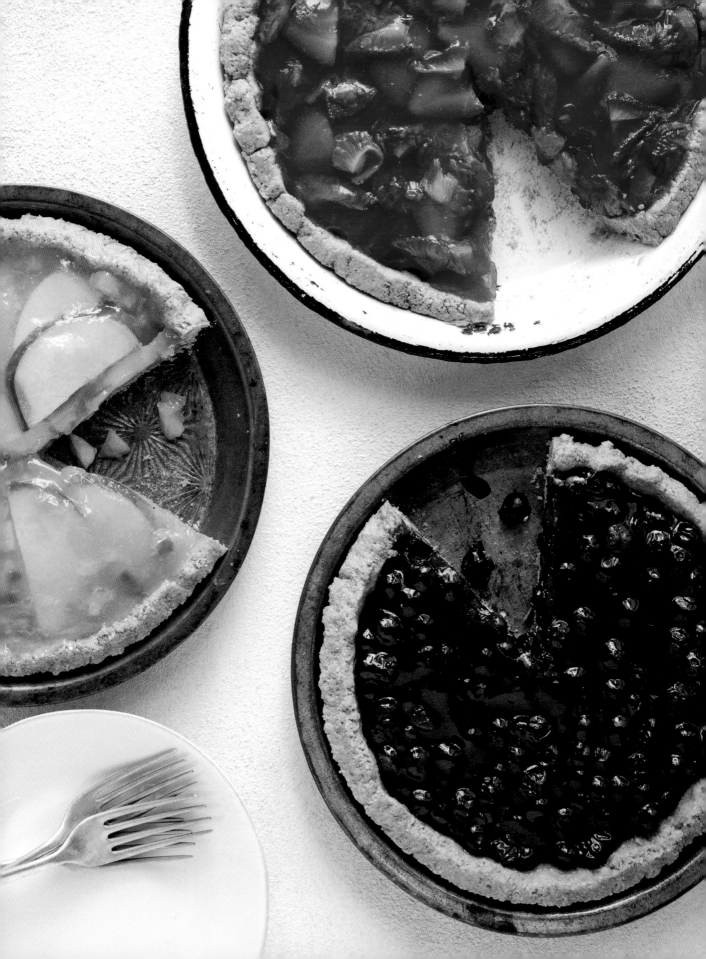

RECIPE INDEX

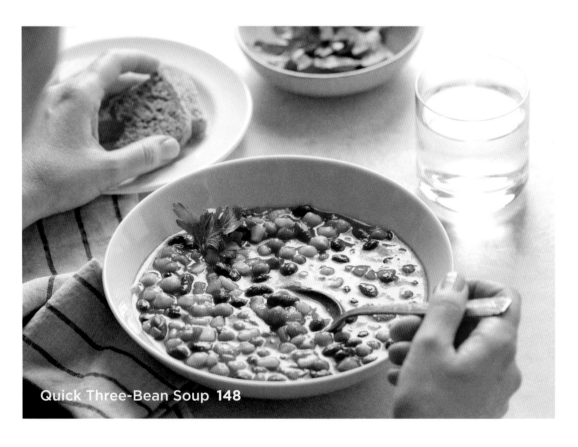

Quick Three-Bean Soup **148**

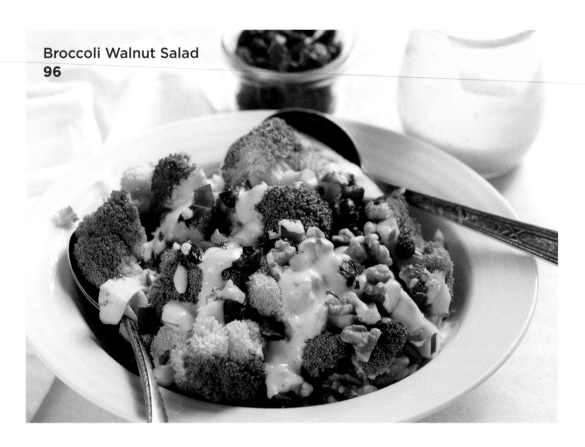

Broccoli Walnut Salad
96

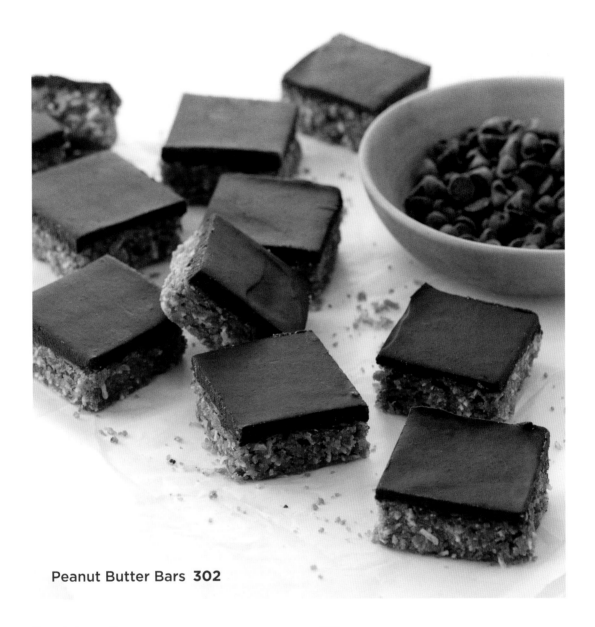

Peanut Butter Bars **302**

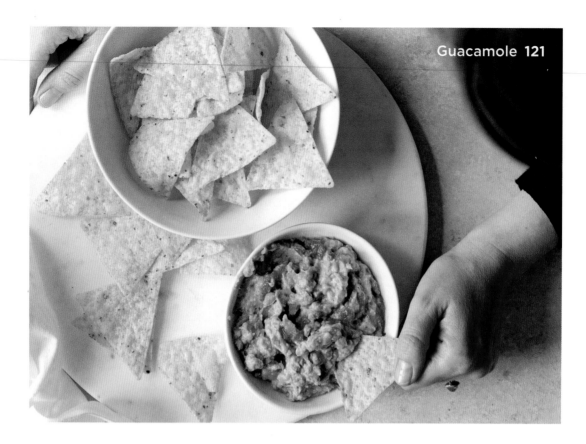

Guacamole **121**

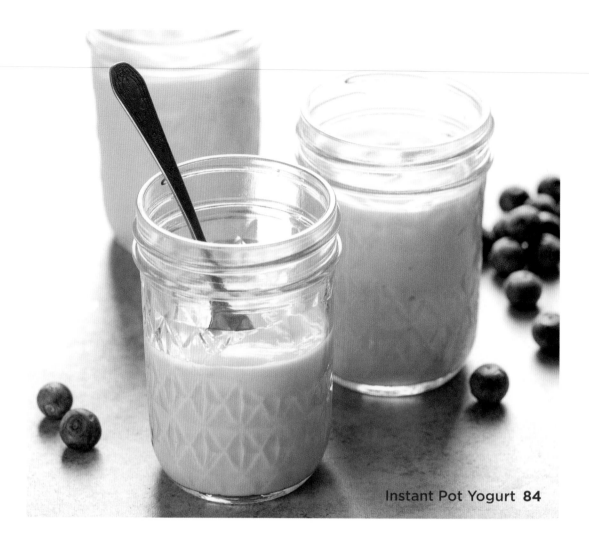

Instant Pot Yogurt **84**

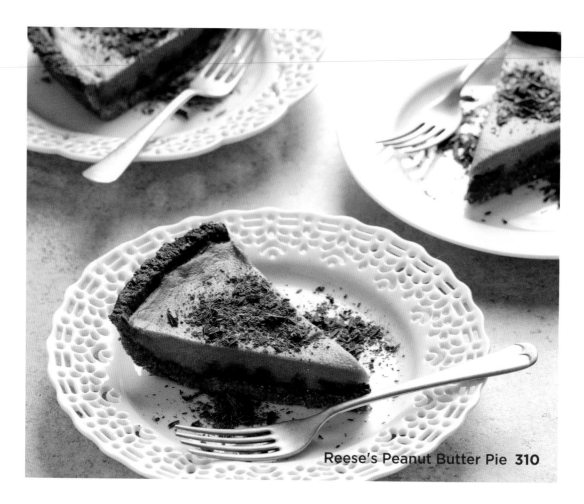

Reese's Peanut Butter Pie **310**

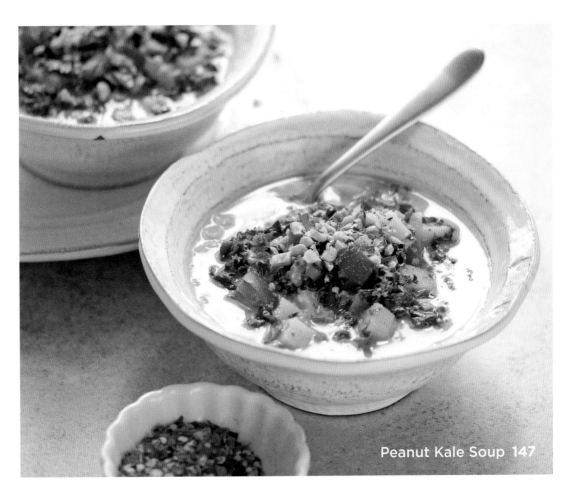

Peanut Kale Soup 147

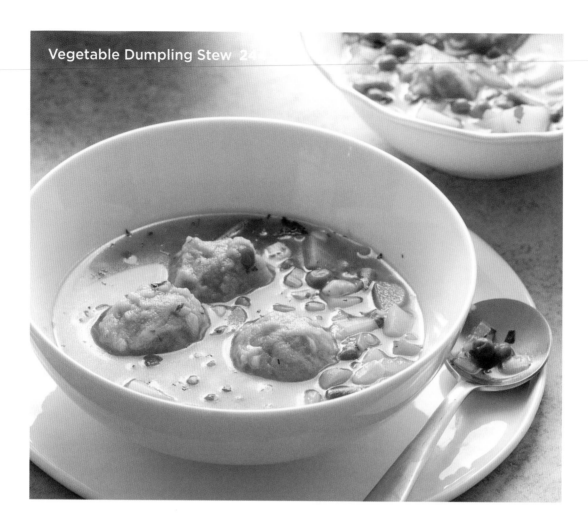

Vegetable Dumpling Stew 244

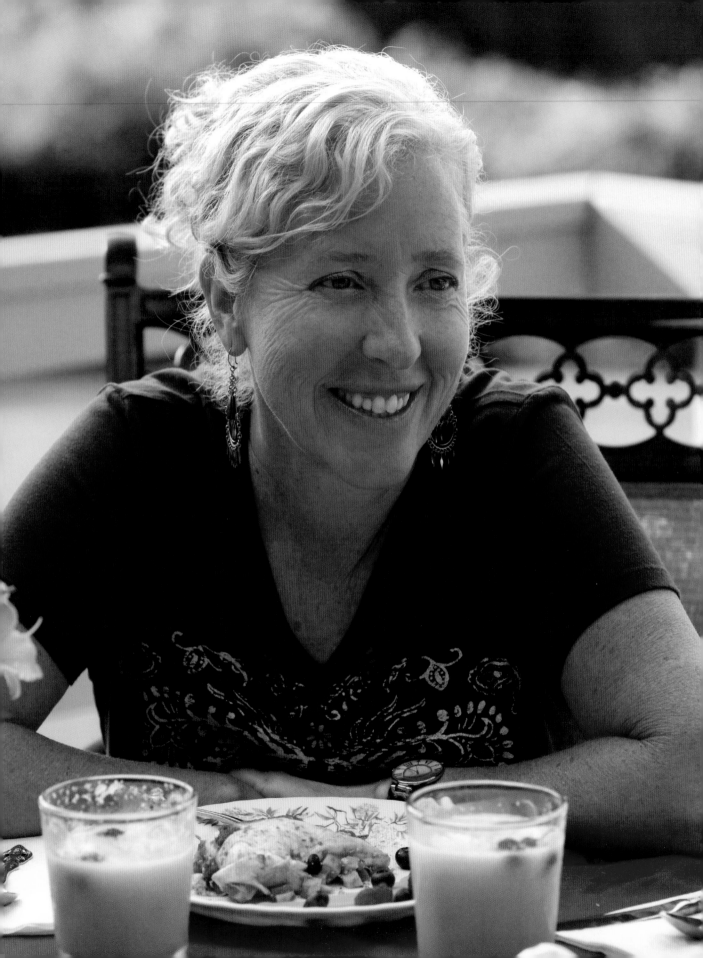

ABOUT THE AUTHOR

LeAnne Campbell, PhD, currently lives in the mountains of La Cumbre, Dominican Republic. She is the president and founder of Global Roots, an organization that fosters the development of healthy, inclusive, and sustainable communities. This is accomplished through community initiatives, conferences, and workshops held at the SOMOS Education Center in La Cumbre. Surrounded by cacao (chocolate) trees, banana, plantain, avocado, coffee, mango, pineapple, jack fruit, cassava, sweet potatoes, and a very lush vegetable garden, she is able to prepare an abundance and variety of whole foods, plant-based meals. She shares the process of harvesting and preparing this food on her website, GlobalRoots.net. LeAnne has more than twenty-five years' experience preparing meals based on a whole foods, plant-based diet and has raised two sons—Steven and Nelson, now twenty-four and twenty-three years old, respectively—on this diet. As a working mother, LeAnne has found ways to prepare quick and easy meals without using animal products or adding oil.

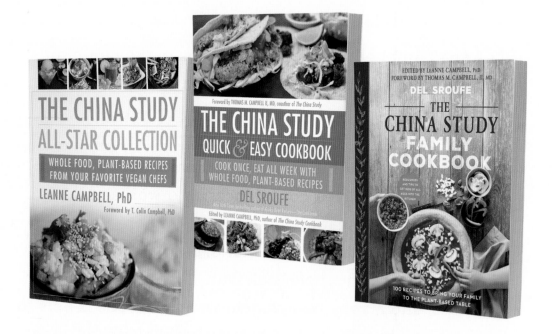
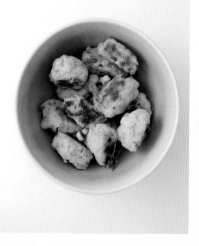
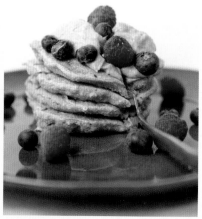
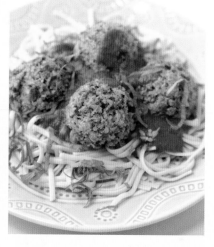

Download a **FREE** digital copy of
*BenBella's Best of
Plant-Based Eating*
and sign up for more
exclusive offers and info at
BENBELLAVEGAN.COM

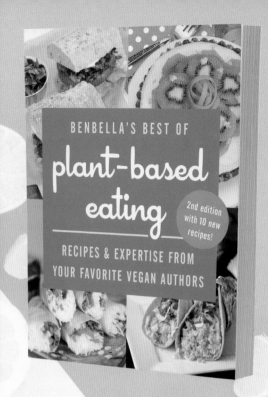

WITH NEARLY 50 RECIPES FROM

The China Study cookbook series
Lindsay S. Nixon's The Happy Herbivore series
Chef Del Sroufe's *Better Than Vegan*
Christy Morgan's *Blissful Bites*
Tracy Russell's *The Best Green Smoothies on the Planet*
Jeff and Joan Stanford's *Dining at The Ravens*
Eric Brent and Glen Merzer's *The HappyCow Cookbook*
Laura Theodore's *Jazzy Vegetarian Classics*
Christina Ross' *Love Fed*
Dreen Burton's *Plant-Powered Families*
Kim Campbell's *The PlantPure Nation Cookbook*
Heather Crosby's *YumUniverse*

AND SELECTIONS FROM

T. Colin Campbell and Howard Jacobsons' *Whole* and *The Low-Carb Fraud*
Dr. Pam Popper and Glen Merzer's *Food Over Medicine*
J. Morris Hicks' *Healthy Eating, Healthy World*
Lani Muelrath's *The Plant-Based Journey*

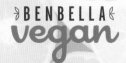